CYSTIC FIBROSIS
A Family Affair

JANE CHUMBLEY is a journalist with wide experience writing for consumer magazines. She also works as an antenatal teacher with the National Childbirth Trust and is in regular contact with couples as they make the transition to parenthood. She contributes regularly to *Practical Parenting* magazine and *Bella* where she used to be the health editor. It was there that she first found out about cystic fibrosis when she met Anne Lovell and her two daughters, Kate and Jo. Since then she has been constantly impressed by their courage, tenacity and dedication to each other as a family.

Acknowledgements

I would like to thank the staff at the Cystic Fibrosis Trust for their practical help with the book, the Family and Adult Support Services workers for their help in recruiting people for me to talk to and – most of all – the parents and young adults with cystic fibrosis who were willing to speak so honestly and at such length.

* denotes that an address or other details are provided in the 'Further information' section.

Overcoming Common Problems

Cystic Fibrosis
A Family Affair

Jane Chumbley

sheldon **PRESS**

First published in Great Britain in 1999 by
Sheldon Press, SPCK, Marylebone Road, London NW1 4DU

Copyright © Jane Chumbley 1999

British Library Cataloguing-in-Publication Data
A catalogue for this book is available from the British Library

ISBN 0–85969–771–1

Typeset by Deltatype Ltd, Birkenhead, Merseyside
Printed in Great Britain by
Biddles Ltd, Guildford and King's Lynn

Contents

Preface

I remember the afternoon in the Children's Outpatients Clinic at University College Hospital, London, where we learned that our first daughter, Kate, and her new-born baby sister, Jo, both had cystic fibrosis. I remember hearing that this was a serious illness that might mean they would not live long and that, because Kate had not been diagnosed before her sister had been conceived, we now had two children with this inherited condition. I remember being told that because we were 'carriers', I should avoid another pregnancy.

I listened to what I was being told and tried to take it in. But I felt numb – and overwhelmed. And I knew that our lives had changed for ever.

We had never heard of cystic fibrosis – and David, their father, went off to the local library to look it up in a medical dictionary. He also found out that there was a charity called the Cystic Fibrosis Trust, which we contacted for information. Our GP came to the house and talked to us one evening – and by chance, some friends we'd met on holiday the previous year knew a couple who had a son with CF. We talked to them on the telephone for hours. But even so, I remember we felt very alone – and afraid. That was in 1972.

So much has changed since then. Parents of a child diagnosed as having cystic fibrosis today have the benefit of all the succeeding years of research, experience in treatment, and the growth and development of the CF Trust and its support services for families.

But until now, there hasn't been one book, like this, which parents can pick up, read from cover to cover, or dip in and out of, and find help, advice, and basic, down-to-earth information about how to live with cystic fibrosis.

I wish that it had been there for us 27 years ago. But I'm extremely glad that it is available from now on.

I'm indebted to Jane Chumbley, a former Health Editor of *Bella*, who agreed to take the project on, and has written such an excellent, practical, clear and concise book for all parents of children with cystic fibrosis.

Knowledge is power – and armed with the wealth of knowledge contained within this book, we can give our children the best chance of survival into adulthood and a positive, hopeful outlook on life as they go through it.

Anne Lovell

Journalist, broadcaster and agony aunt at *Bella* magazine

Foreword

As Chief Executive of the Cystic Fibrosis Trust, I feel for families and individuals coping with this distressing, complex and poorly understood disease. So it is refreshing indeed to read an account of Cystic Fibrosis which is so human, so clear and so comprehensive. All aspects of life with Cystic Fibrosis are explored in an honest and positive way. Not only will readers be better informed, they will have the comfort of hearing of the experiences of others. To know you are not alone in facing a problem does make it easier to cope.

Individuals from all walks of life are linked by the common experience of being affected by Cystic Fibrosis and they do take enormous comfort from knowing they are supported by 'the Cystic Fibrosis family'. *Cystic Fibrosis – A Family Affair* captures the essence of the hopes and fears of so many families, and reflects the reality of living with such a serious condition.

Families newly coping with Cystic Fibrosis, as well as those who have lived with it for years, will take great comfort from this book. For those not affected directly, the book offers a compassionate and moving glimpse into the resilience and strength that so many of us find we have when faced with great adversity.

Above all, it offers real hope and shows the way to live life to the full, even when coping with a life threatening illness.

Rosie Barnes
Chief Executive
Cystic Fibrosis Trust

Introduction

'It was awful. It was the worst thing that ever could have happened. I just went into a daze and kept thinking this isn't happening. You feel like someone's cheated on you. Later on I used to see other babies and think why couldn't it have been them? Why me?'

Your child has cystic fibrosis. Even as you read this you may be in shock: stunned by the news that your child has a condition for which there is currently no cure. Your mind may be reeling with all sorts of questions. How could this happen? What does it mean? What can we do? Or you may feel quite, quite numb – as though none of this is really happening and you are watching yourself in a dream. You may feel completely helpless and very confused. Only one thing is certain: life will never be the same again. As one mother said:

'When your child has CF it's like you enter a different world. You have to learn all about these things you never knew about before, and you see things differently.'

Cystic fibrosis affects the whole family and all the relationships within it. Parents often say there isn't an hour that goes by when they don't think about CF. That kind of pressure is bound to have an effect on the way you interact with your partner, the way you respond to your other children and – of course – the way you behave when you are with your child who has CF. Grandparents, aunts and uncles and the wider family are also caught up in the ripple effect as the news spreads and they come to terms with what it could mean for them personally. Because it is a genetic disorder, cystic fibrosis truly is a family affair.

How to use this book

You have probably bought, borrowed or even been given this book because your child or a close relative has been diagnosed as having CF. When you're first given news of this kind it's very hard to take in what you're told. Suddenly you've entered a new world that you previously knew nothing about: a world of physiotherapy, enzymes and antibiotics. A world where people sometimes use terms you don't fully understand,

and where you may suddenly feel very cut off from your friends. It's hard to take in what's happened, let alone the implications and the information which you will need to help you cope with CF.

The specialist teams who work with the parents of children with CF understand this only too well. They will give you time and patiently explain when you ask questions. No one expects you to remember everything straightaway, or to become an overnight expert in CF. After all, it's a unique and very complicated condition. The staff at the Cystic Fibrosis Trust* are there to help you, with local support workers and local groups of ordinary people who have been through this already.

This book is here to supplement the work these people do. It offers background information which will help you to reach a deeper under-standing of CF – if that's what you want. It also offers you the opportunity to hear from a wide range of people whose children have CF or who have CF themselves. You can benefit from their experience, their advice and from the knowledge that other people feel the same way as you: your feelings are perfectly normal.

You may also be reading this book as the parent of a teenager or young adult with CF, or because you yourself are growing up with CF. You may have a sense that life is changing for you, that you are moving into uncharted territory and feel that you need some information and a chance to think through your feelings. The second part of the book should help with this.

Whatever your situation, you might want to read the book cover to cover. On the other hand, it has been written so you can dip in and out. Right now you may be desperate for information on living with CF. Later on you might want to read how other couples have coped and kept their relationship strong despite the strain CF can place on a family. You can also use the book to check on individual words or phrases you've heard used. The book will never take the place of detailed discussions with the team caring for your child: they are the experts in CF.

Three parts

The book is divided into three parts. Part one is a guide for parents whose child has been diagnosed with cystic fibrosis. It looks at living with CF, the daily treatment routines, the kind of care you can expect from health professionals and the impact CF has on couples and families. It starts with a very detailed explanation of CF, and a section answering the questions bewildered parents sometimes ask. You may want to skip over some of this detail – it certainly isn't essential reading, but some people feel the need for a deeper understanding.

Part two looks at life for young adults who have CF. If your child has been recently diagnosed as having CF this section may not seem immediately relevant to you, but at the back of your mind you may have lots of questions about your child's long-term future. What are people with CF able to do? How do they cope during the adolescent years? What is it like to grow up knowing your life could be shortened? Does the condition change in adult years? The good news is that although your child has a serious condition, college, university, professional jobs, homes and families are all possible.

The second chapter of Part two focuses on the emotional and practical implications of your son or daughter's progression from child to adolescent and adult. It will be difficult to judge when to let go of the responsibility you have carried for so long, but there will come a time when your child is able to do her own physio or administer his own drugs. And it will be hard not to be over-protective. In this chapter parents and young people talk honestly about their struggles to separate and yet remain close.

The remaining chapter of Part two looks at specific issues which young adults with CF have to face these days: leaving home, getting a mortgage and insurance, relationships, fertility treatments, and getting a job. Obviously a lot of this may change in the future.

Part three looks at the prospect of new treatments for CF and the progress of research into gene therapy. Research into such a complex disorder is bound to appear painstakingly slow to onlookers and people who want new treatments to be available quickly, but scientists working on CF are making very real progress in discovering more about the condition, which is the important first step in developing those new treatments.

The book finishes on a very positive note: there's no denying that the diagnosis of CF is a body blow, and it does take time to come to terms with what is happening to your family. But the prospects are so much better than they were even ten years ago and in ten years' time they will be even better still. People with CF can and do live long, productive and fulfilling lives. As one mother said:

'It does get easier. The shock wears off, you come down to earth and you get on with it. You don't ever come to terms with it and nothing ever gets back to normal, but you do learn to live with it.'

PART ONE

Finding out

1

What is cystic fibrosis?

'Like most parents, I suppose, I'd heard of CF but I didn't know exactly what it was. You just don't go into these things do you?'

Cystic fibrosis is a genetic disorder. Put simply, cystic fibrosis or CF occurs because of a fault in one of the genes we inherit from our parents. CF is not something you catch or develop, it's a condition you're born with, although in some cases it can take months or even years for the symptoms to develop to the point where it is suspected and diagnosed. Estimates suggest that about one in four children with CF is more than 18 months old when the diagnosis is finally made. A very small number of people are diagnosed when they are adults.

If your child has CF it is important to understand how the condition is inherited because this may have implications for future pregnancies. It is also helpful background for understanding the new 'gene therapy' which is being researched at the moment.

Genetics for beginners

Every cell in your body contains 23 pairs of chromosomes. One of each pair of chromosomes is inherited from your father and one from your mother. Each chromosome is like a string, attached to which are literally thousands of genes – tiny pieces of DNA. Each gene has a specific job to do, making a particular protein which determines how something in your body works. So, for example, there is a gene which determines the colour of your eyes and another which controls blood-clotting. One of the genes on chromosome 7 controls the way water and salts pass in and out of cells in the body.

The chromosomes have been compared to a set of thick instruction manuals in which each gene is a single paragraph. When a gene is defective or faulty it's as if something has been misspelt so the instructions can't be read. In practice, the faulty gene makes a faulty protein that can prevent some bodily function working properly.

Like chromosomes, genes are paired: one of each pair is inherited from the mother and the other from the father. In a few genetic disorders, a single faulty gene from either the mother or the father is enough to cause the disease, even if the paired gene inherited from the other parent is perfectly normal. This is called *dominant* inheritance – because the faulty gene is dominant.

In other conditions, the disorder only occurs if a child gets a pair of faulty genes – one from each parent. This is called *recessive* inheritance – because the faulty gene is hidden until it pairs up with another faulty gene. With recessive conditions, you can have a single faulty gene and know absolutely nothing about it because the normal gene compensates and gets the job done.

Genetics and cystic fibrosis

Cystic fibrosis is caused by a pair of faulty genes on chromosome 7 – the genes responsible for controlling the way water and salts pass in and out of cells in the body. CF is a recessive condition. In other words, to get it you have to inherit the CF gene from your mother *and* your father. It is important that all the family understand this when a child is diagnosed with CF. Sometimes grandparents can say particularly hurtful things – implying, for example, that the CF must have come from the other side because 'there's never been anything like that in our family'. But the CF gene *must* come from both sides if someone has the condition.

Of course, it is perfectly possible that there has never been anyone with cystic fibrosis on your side, or indeed either side of the family within living memory, but the faulty gene was there nevertheless – being carried by completely healthy and unknowing individuals. This is possible because the condition is recessive. If you inherit a single CF gene on one chromosome 7 and a normal gene on the other chromosome 7 then you are a carrier and CF carriers have no symptoms of cystic fibrosis at all: the normal gene compensates.

The bottom line is that both parents must have the faulty gene and both must pass it on before a baby inherits CF. Figure 1 below illustrates how this could happen. If only one parent is a carrier it is impossible for the child to have CF, although he or she may inherit the faulty gene and become a carrier too.

Statistically speaking, the chances of two CF carriers having a child with CF is one in four (see Figure 1). There is a one-in-two chance their child will be a carrier, and a one-in-four chance the child won't inherit any faulty CF genes.

This doesn't mean that if you have four children only one of them will have CF. That's possible, but in reality the risks are the same for each pregnancy. So if you've already had one child with CF it doesn't mean

4

future children are any more or less likely to inherit the condition – the risk is one in four for each pregnancy where the partners both carry CF.

The cystic fibrosis gene

The CF gene was actually identified in 1989, although scientists had known for many years that it existed. Normally the gene produces a protein called CFTR – cystic fibrosis transmembrane conductance

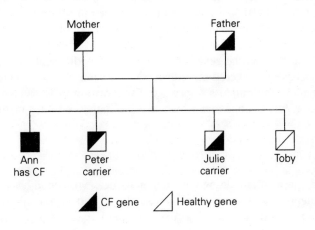

Ann has CF because she has inherited two CF genes – one from her mother and one from her father.

Peter is a CF carrier because although he has inherited a normal gene from his father he has inherited a CF gene from his mother.

Julie is also a CF carrier since she has inherited a CF gene from her father along with a normal gene from her mother.

Toby doesn't have CF and isn't a carrier because he has inherited two normal genes – one from his father and one from his mother.

Figure 1: Diagram illustrating how the CF gene can be passed on by two carriers

regulator – which works a bit like a valve or pump, carrying sodium, chloride and water in and out of the cells lining the lungs and the digestive tract (the oesophagus and the intestines). This is a bit hard to imagine, but the protein sits in the membrane or outer layer of the cells which line the lungs and most other parts of the body and is a bit like a tube with a pump and an on/off switch. The pump and the switch control how much salt and water pass out of the cell.

The faulty CF gene may fail to produce any CFTR protein, it may produce a dud version where the pump doesn't switch on and off properly (so it doesn't let out enough water and the mucus on the outside of the cell gets too thick) or it may produce CFTR which isn't transported properly to the cell membrane. This last defect or mutation is called delta F508 – a name which describes to scientists the place where the CFTR protein is damaged. About four out of five people with CF have this kind of gene defect. Occasionally, however, there are other mutations and the gene is faulty in a slightly different way. So far scientists have discovered more than 600 mutations, most of them very rare. Some of the mutations appear to cause a form of CF which leads to fewer complications and which may be diagnosed later in life.

Getting a diagnosis

The fact that you're reading this book may mean your child has already been diagnosed as having cystic fibrosis. Ideally doctors should explain how they have reached that diagnosis but even if they do, the explanation may be hard to take in at the time. Your mind may be reeling with the implications of the diagnosis, not necessarily how it was made. On the other hand, your instinct may be to ask 'Are you sure?', to doubt the diagnosis, and to want proof. Whichever way you react, it can be helpful to know more about the tests which are done to screen for cystic fibrosis.

The Guthrie heel-prick test

In the UK all babies are offered a routine heel-prick test when they are about six days old. The blood sample taken in this way is tested in a lab for rare blood disorders such as haemophilia where the blood does not clot properly. It is possible to test for cystic fibrosis in this way, since levels of a chemical – immunoreactive trypsin – are high in babies with CF. But at this point in time very few health authorities do the test. If your baby was diagnosed as having CF as a result of the Guthrie test that could be seen as a positive sign that people take the condition seriously in your area. There are very real advantages to having an early diagnosis and your baby will benefit from having antibiotics to prevent and quickly treat chest infections which could otherwise do permanent damage to the developing lungs. A recent study showed that nearly one in three one-month-old babies with CF already had signs of an infection.

A so-called 'positive' result in this test – in other words, one where there are signs the baby may have CF – should always be followed up with further tests: a sweat test (see below) and a DNA test on a blood sample to confirm the faulty CF genes.

Sweat test

Although children with CF do not sweat more than other children, their sweat contains more salt than normal. Some parents say they notice when kissing their child that he or she tastes a bit salty. The sweat test involves collecting sweat over a period of time and measuring the amount of salt it contains. There are several different ways of doing this – heating the skin on an arm or leg, for example, and then collecting the sweat produced in the next 10–30 minutes. The tests are completely painless and don't damage the child's skin in any way, but the results aren't always clear-cut and the test may need repeating. Normally you'd expect to find salt (sodium and chloride) in concentrations of 15–30 mmol per litre. In children with CF the concentration is likely to be greater than 70 mmol per litre.

It is standard practice to follow up a high result with a DNA test on a blood sample which can confirm the diagnosis.

The sweat test is used to follow up the signs or symptoms which suggest CF, including: the findings of a Guthrie test; a newborn baby having a bowel obstruction (see below); a child having repeated chest infections; a long-standing cough; constant diarrhoea or low weight gain; or another child in the family being confirmed as having CF.

Prenatal diagnosis

This involves testing the unborn baby for CF early in pregnancy. Chapter 4 contains details of the tests available.

'Ellen had been ill since she was three weeks old. She was in and out of hospital all the time and the doctors said she had pneumonia and kept sending her home with antibiotics. She had a nasty barking cough and from ten weeks on, every time she fed she vomited and she never gained any weight. Eventually when she was five months old and weighed only 8lb they did the sweat test and discovered she had CF.'

'I was breastfeeding Peter but he wasn't gaining much weight so at ten weeks they suggested I put him onto solids and it was then we realised something was wrong: he was in constant pain, his stools were soft and the doctor referred us to the hospital for tests. We tried various diets and had two sweat tests, but they were both negative. They thought for a long time he was coeliac but he just got thinner and thinner and more and more poorly. Eventually when he was 19 months old they sent us to Great Ormond Street where they did a sweat test with the proper equipment and discovered he was CF after all. As a result the local hospital got the proper equipment to do the sweat test. I did doubt the diagnosis a bit because his chest was always so good and he did so well on his diet. He was always so fit and healthy. I thought perhaps he's only got it mildly or something – I didn't really understand at first. But he's had more chest infections since he's got older.'

'Robert was a big baby when he was born – 9lb 4oz – but he didn't put on much, he was sick all the time and he had smelly poo. Then he had a nasty cough. The GP said it was asthma but it carried on and in the end when he was four months we asked if we could go to the hospital. The doctor there asked lots of questions about his cough, his weight, his poo and whether he tasted salty. Then they did the test for CF and called me to say he'd got it.'

'They said they were going to do the test and I didn't think anything of it. Then I told one of the nurses when I was in the kitchen making up a bottle and I asked "Can they die of it?" and she said "Yes". Just like that. And my whole world fell apart. But later on, after we'd got the result, the health visitor came round and she was fantastic. She put it all into perspective.'

'Andrew was two years old when they eventually diagnosed CF. My wife had been going bananas washing stained nappies and there were a number of little things we were anxious about, but my wife was basically labelled as a neurotic mother. He was sent home originally with low birthweight and jaundice, but nothing was picked up. We just seemed to be going to the doctor's a lot. We kept badgering them until they eventually did a sweat test. Even then the paediatrician was trying to tell us it was coeliac disease.'

Symptoms which suggest CF in a baby or young child:
- persistent cough;
- bouts of coughing ending in vomiting;
- phlegm in vomit;
- wheezing, particularly after coughing or exercising;
- repeated chest infections;
- failure to gain weight;
- blocked nose;
- pale, fatty, bulky, smelly poo;
- swollen abdomen with skinny arms and legs;
- sweat tastes salty;
- prolapsed rectum (see below);
- blocked bowel (see below).

What does CF mean for my child?

The fact that the CF gene doesn't allow enough water to escape from the cells means that the cell secretions are much thicker and stickier than normal. Most of the lining surfaces in the body contain cells which secrete and all of them are potentially affected by CF. In practice, the greatest problems are seen in the lungs and the pancreas, but the salivary glands, the intestine and the gall bladder can all get clogged up or obstructed.

Digestion

The pancreas is a gland in the abdomen which links up with the small intestine. It has two main jobs to do – producing chemicals called insulin and glucagon which control the amount of sugar in the blood, and producing digestive juices called pancreatic enzymes which pass into the small intestine. Along with bile salts produced in the gall bladder, these enzymes help to break down the fat, proteins and carbohydrate we eat so that they can be easily absorbed. The pancreas also secretes bicarbonate which helps to neutralize stomach acid and so allows the enzymes to do their job.

Although people with CF usually have enough insulin, the digestive juices can get blocked by the sticky mucus building up in the channels that lead to the intestine and there isn't enough bicarbonate to reduce stomach acidity. In practice this means two things: first the pancreas develops cysts and fibrous, gristly tissue. Second, fat in the diet isn't absorbed properly which explains why some babies with CF fail to gain weight and have fatty, bulky or very runny bowel motions. Not everyone with CF is affected this badly, however. It is estimated that around one in ten people with CF get at least some enzymes from their pancreas. Some people seem to get plenty and have very few, if any, digestive problems. These people almost certainly have a different mutation on the faulty gene.

Children with CF may also be short of important fat-soluble vitamins and minerals as these are also absorbed with the help of pancreatic juices.

Chapter 2 explains the importance of the trace vitamins and minerals and how taking enzyme supplements with meals helps to counter the digestive problems and malnutrition caused by CF.

Coughs, chest infections and breathing

The lungs contain a network of hollow tubes a bit like the branches of a tree. The major branches – the bronchi – lead to smaller branches and twigs – the bronchioles. The air which you breathe in is taken down this network of tubes to reach tiny air sacs or alveoli where oxygen is passed into the blood and carbon dioxide removed so that it can be breathed out. All the tubes are lined with mucus-secreting cells and fine hairs called cilia. The mucus and hairs work together to keep the tubes clear: if particles of dust or bacteria are breathed in they get lodged in the mucus and are wafted upwards by the cilia to the larger passages where they can be coughed up or swallowed.

Babies with CF have perfectly normal lungs when they are born, but the mucus produced in them is unusually thick which means the cilia can't move it upwards and the natural lung-cleaning process is halted. This explains why young children with CF tend to wheeze, struggle to breathe and cough a lot as they try to clear their lungs. Without treatment, some of the bronchioles, the smaller tubes, can get blocked and can be infected by bacteria and viruses which aren't being cleared out. If bacteria build up in the mucus, the lining of the tubes becomes swollen and the tubes may react by producing more mucus to get rid of the bacteria, leading to infection. These infections can cause scarring and permanent damage in the lungs.

That's why children with CF need a combination of physiotherapy to clear the sticky mucus and antibiotics to prevent chest infections (see chapter 2). But there's more to infection than the failure of the normal mucus clearing system:

- Researchers have discovered that cells in the lung affected by CF make only small quantities of chemicals involved in producing nitric oxide (an anti-bacterial agent which helps to fight infection – see chapter 9 for more details).
- Scientists also believe that the cells lining the lungs of people with CF produce receptors – like attractive landing sites – to which bacteria attach. These receptors increase in number as lung damage progresses, setting up a vicious cycle of infections causing more damage.
- The body's natural protective anti-bacterial chemicals – called defensins – are also neutralized by the high levels of salt in lungs affected by CF.

New drug treatments are being developed which might, in the future, counter some of these problems (see chapter 9).

As well as coughing and suffering from chest infections, about one in three children with CF have asthma on and off – wheezing and finding it difficult to breathe as the tiny airways in the lungs become narrowed. Asthma is treated with drugs which relax and open the airways. These drugs can be delivered using a nebulizer or an inhaler.

The rest of the body

Bowels

About one in ten babies born with CF is very ill in the first few days with a bowel obstruction. The most common form of obstruction is called meconium ileus: the meconium – the thick, black substance which lines the normal unborn baby's gut – is so thick and sticky in the baby with CF that it blocks the bowel. Meconium ileus causes vomiting and a swollen abdomen. Babies with meconium ileus need an urgent operation to bypass and relieve the blockage or – more often these days – to remove the blocked part of the bowel.

'Our first son had meconium ileus when he was born and he was kept in hospital for four months although he didn't need surgery. I thought there was no chance my second son would have it as well but he did, and he needed major surgery. They actually removed several inches of his intestine, but they're now aged 29 and 25 and

11

have been very healthy!' (Susan, mother of Peter and John who both have CF)

Older children and adults with CF may suffer from meconium ileus equivalent or distal intestinal obstruction syndrome (respectively known as MIE or DIOS for short) where the bowel gets blocked with mucus and fatty stools and causes pain and vomiting. The problem can usually be treated by increasing the amount of enzymes being taken with meals, and with drugs which help to thin the mucus in the intestine. There's no connection between meconium ileus at birth and MIE later in life.

Neonatal jaundice

Jaundice (yellowing of the skin and the whites of the eyes) is very common in newborn babies and usually resolves on its own without any treatment. A few need light treatment (phototherapy) to break down the excess bilirubin pigment in the skin which is causing the yellowing. But newborn babies with CF may sometimes have prolonged jaundice, perhaps because of mucus in the bile channels which slows down the rate at which bilirubin can be excreted from the body. Even so, the jaundice usually resolves in time and isn't dangerous unless the levels of bilirubin get very high. Babies who are jaundiced are monitored to ensure this doesn't happen.

Stomach aches

These are a bit of a mystery complication since no one is exactly sure why children with CF have tummy aches – it may be something to do with coughing or the amount of enzymes they are taking with meals. A sharp abdominal pain is different, however, especially if your child is vomiting as well: this could be the result of an intussusception – a piece of the bowel starts folding in on itself, a bit like a child's toy telescope. If this isn't treated, blood vessels start being dragged into the fold, and the blood supply to the bowel can be blocked, leading to gangrene. This is something that can happen to anyone – it's not exclusive to people with CF – but it is quite rare, particularly in children. Obviously it's a surgical emergency and needs urgent attention in hospital.

Rectal prolapse

Part of the lining of the rectum slips out of the anus, probably because it has been weakened by the amount of bulky poo that has gone through it. This generally only happens with very young children and it can make them feel as though they need to do a poo, although it often happens after they've been straining to do a poo in the first place. It can also happen after a bout of coughing. A rectal prolapse isn't usually painful although it can be a bit worrying when you see it for the first time. Usually it goes back on its own: you just need to get your child to lie down and relax if possible – you could both lie down on the bed and read a book, for example. If it doesn't go back in then you may need to push it in, and the first time this happens it's worth contacting your GP for help.

Nasal polyps

These are growths in the mucous membrane lining the nose. If necessary they can be removed surgically, but they tend to recur.

Older children and adults with CF may find the condition affects other parts of the body including the liver, the joints, the heart, the sinuses and the reproductive system. About one in ten adults with CF also develops a mild form of diabetes. Chapter 6 contains more details of these complications.

If you've read all through this section you may be feeling horrified. But the truth is that your child may not suffer any of these complications. At this stage, no one can say exactly what CF will mean for your child. Some children are very, very ill until their routine CF treatment gets underway and then they are fine for many, many years. These days, many children who are diagnosed at a young age can expect to be healthy until their late teens:

> 'Her stomach had shrunk so much that a month after CF was diagnosed she was back in hospital for drip feeds. But that was six years ago, and she hasn't been in hospital since.' (Judy, mother of Ellen aged seven)

Questions and answers

Can cystic fibrosis be cured?

No – at least, not at the moment. The treatments for CF – including physiotherapy, enzymes, antibiotics, and nasal sprays – are aimed at minimizing the symptoms and side effects of the condition: they won't cure it. However, scientists are working on new approaches including gene therapy which may in the future offer the prospect of a partial cure (see below and chapter 9).

Is there a way to replace the faulty gene that causes cystic fibrosis?
In theory this sounds like the solution, doesn't it? In practice, replacing
a gene – a tiny piece of genetic material – is incredibly complicated.
But scientists are working on it. Most of the gene therapy techniques
which are being developed at the moment are aimed at trying to transfer
the normal gene into the lungs. That won't solve the problems caused in
the pancreas or elsewhere in the body but it could make life a lot easier
for people with CF. Chapter 9 has more details about the latest research
into new treatments.

Does CF affect more girls than boys?
No. There is no evidence to suggest that gender has anything to do with
the chances of inheriting two copies of the faulty gene. CF affects girls
and boys in equal numbers.

Is cystic fibrosis a new condition?
No. It has been around for a long time but it was only fully recognized
in the 1930s. In those days children with CF didn't live very long
because they weren't given the antibiotics which fight chest infections.
In fact, seven out of ten died before they were a year old.

How common is cystic fibrosis?
More common than a lot of people think. In fact, CF is the most
common life-threatening inherited disease in the UK. About one in
2,500 babies born here has CF – that's about 250 babies a year or five a
week. It is estimated that there are currently around 6,500 people with
CF in the UK, between a third and a half of them over 15 years old. It is
very likely the number of adults with CF will go on increasing as
people are living for longer as a result of improved treatments.

The CF gene itself is very widespread: around two million people in
the UK are carriers – that's about one in 25 of us. But most carriers will
have no idea they have the gene because they are perfectly well.
Carrying the gene is only significant if you have children with another
carrier, or if you pass the gene onto your children who then have
children with another carrier.

Could the diagnosis be wrong?
Probably not, but sweat tests aren't like pregnancy tests, they don't give
you a yes/no answer. In practice, your child won't have been given a
sweat test unless there were other symptoms which suggested cystic
fibrosis was a possibility, so the results of a sweat test are never seen in

isolation. If your child had a borderline result in the sweat test – in other words, if the concentration of salt in the sweat was high, but not that high – then the test should be repeated twice. And all positive sweat tests should be followed up with a blood test. The sweat test needs to be done very carefully and by someone experienced. Ideally it should be done in one of the large specialist centres. If you have any doubts about the result of your test, contact the Cystic Fibrosis Trust* for information about the specialist centres in your area.

Why wasn't my child diagnosed sooner?
It is very difficult to answer this question. Some NHS Trusts and health authorities have decided not to include cystic fibrosis in the range of conditions they screen for in the Guthrie test. In many cases this is a purely financial decision, a fact which is probably hard for you to come to terms with if you feel your child has suffered permanent lung damage because she wasn't diagnosed quickly. The fact is that without this kind of screening, CF is only picked up when a child has recurrent infections and other signs such as diarrhoea and poor weight gain. Even when all these symptoms are present it's possible doctors might not think to test for CF and if that's your experience then again it's natural to feel angry or bitter. If your child has been diagnosed late – after 18 months, for example – it may be because he or she has a milder form of CF.

It may be important to acknowledge your anger, to talk to the doctors involved and to get information about how the diagnosis was made. You may even want an independent doctor to review your child's notes. Unfortunately, it's impossible to turn back the clock. The most important thing is to get the best possible treatment now the condition has been diagnosed. If you have lost confidence in your GP, or the doctors treating your child, then you may want to change consultant, GP or hospital. Chapter 3 contains advice about getting the best possible care and information about the various roles played by your GP, the local hospital and specialist centres.

Why has this happened to us?
You could say it's purely a matter of chance, and a remote chance at that. If it's true that one in 25 people carry the CF gene then there's roughly a one-in-625 chance that two carriers will become partners $(1/25 \times 1/25 = 1/625)$. After that, there's a one-in-four chance your child will have CF. That's an overall chance of one in 2,500.

Why is it called cystic fibrosis?

The name cystic fibrosis comes from early reports about the condition and refers to the damage seen in the pancreas. This consists of cysts and fibrosis – scarring and thickening which leaves gristly tissue behind. CF is also sometimes known as mucoviscidosis because the mucus in the lungs and pancreas is thick and sticky.

My baby had meconium ileus. Does that mean she will be severely affected with CF?

No. In fact, some research suggests the outlook may be slightly better for babies who have survived meconium ileus because it means CF is diagnosed so early on.

Will my child be a midget?

No. In the past a lot of people with CF were below average in height, but these days, with improved understanding about nutrition, your child could grow quite normally. Many parents say that if you looked at a classroom full of similar aged children there's no way you could pick out their child as the one suffering from CF. Adults with CF can be strong, muscular and athletic looking, particularly if they work hard at their fitness.

Why do my other children have to be tested when they are perfectly healthy?

Because CF can be mild in some people, an older child could have the condition hidden for many years. This is relatively unlikely, but it's not unheard of. In one recent case it wasn't until a couple's three-month-old baby was diagnosed with CF that their five-year-old son was tested and found to have CF as well.

What is the outlook for people with cystic fibrosis?

These days, as a result of improved treatment, about three out of four babies with CF survive to adolescence. Increasing numbers survive well into adulthood. People with CF aged 40 and 50 took part in a survey of CF adults in 1994, and there are reports that the oldest person with CF on record was 72 when he died. Since the CF gene was isolated in 1989 there has been dramatic progress in research. The rate of progress with both drug and gene therapy is such that there seems to be a realistic prospect of a cure within your child's lifetime.

2

Living with cystic fibrosis

'You constantly have to balance quality of life and longevity – and you never really know if you've got it right.'

There is no point denying that CF will have a huge impact on daily life for you and your child. Suddenly there seems a lot to learn, a lot of routines to put into place and a lot of changes for you all to cope with. It may help to tackle one thing at a time or for you and your partner to take responsibility for different things – so you each become 'expert' in one area and then share your knowledge together. So, for example, you could take charge of giving pancreatin and any other drugs, and your partner could do the physio to start with. Before long you will both need to be fully aware of the care your child needs, but this division of labour can help you to focus and feel you are getting to grips with something in the early days. It is important to get as much help as you can from the team looking after your child. Ask questions, get on the phone and make all the appointments you need so that you feel reassured you understand what is going on.

The impact of CF on your daily life will depend to some extent on the age of your child at diagnosis and whether you have other children. If you have been used to taking your toddler to the normal clinics and mother and baby groups then you probably already have routines and a number of friends or acquaintances with children of a similar age. There is no reason why you can't carry on as normal so far as these activities are concerned, and it can help you and your child if you keep to your routine. If your baby is only a couple of months old then very few routines are already in place and everything is new. Your baby's needs are very special but in most respects they are exactly the same as those of any other baby and you will benefit from meeting other parents with babies of the same age – at the normal health visitor clinics or at drop-in baby groups. You will still have to make the same decisions about baby equipment, dummies and sleeping arrangements as anyone else. These things aren't affected by the fact your child has CF.

So far as immunizations are concerned, experts advise that children with and without CF respond in the same way. In other words, CF doesn't increase the risk of adverse reaction. So, on the one hand, your decision about this is much the same as for other parents. On the other hand, the childhood infectious diseases can be very nasty and could be risky for

17

children with CF, so if you are inclined not to have the immunizations it is important to discuss this with the doctors involved in caring for your child.

Medication

Most children with CF have at least two sorts of drugs – pancreatic enzymes (pancreatin) and vitamins. Some also take antibiotics to prevent as well as to treat infection. The timing of some drugs has to be linked with the routine physiotherapy. For example, antibiotics should be given after physio, when the lungs have less mucus in them.

Preventive antibiotics

The aim of antibiotic therapy is to prevent the infections which can cause permanent damage to the lungs. It has been established through research that very young babies are vulnerable to bacterial infection, so the earlier antibiotic treatment can begin, the better. Drugs commonly used are flucloxacillin and amoxycillin (Augmentin is one of the brand names) which are penicillin drugs. For children this is usually just one spoonful a day. Other people have nebulized antibiotics every day (see box below). But not all children need – or are offered – routine antibiotics to take every day. Karen's four-year-old son Robert, for example, manages without:

> 'He's not on any preventive medicine. He does get some chest infections, but not very often. Two weeks on antibiotics and it's over and done with. Now he's at school he has started to pick things up, but not loads. He's really quite healthy and as bright as a button.'

Antibiotics for infections

If your child develops a cough then it should be taken seriously. Usually your doctor will prescribe something straightaway while a sample of spit or a swab from the mouth is tested to work out the bacteria involved and the antibiotic which is likely to be most effective. It may be necessary to switch to a different antibiotic when the results of these tests are known. These specific antibiotics can be given as liquid, tablets or capsules or they can be nebulized so that they are inhaled as a mist (see box below).

IV antibiotics

IV stands for intravenous, which means into a vein. If intravenous antibiotics are needed to treat a more serious infection, then a younger child will need to go into hospital, although you can learn how to give the drugs yourself after a line has been inserted into the vein. Having a line put in can be uncomfortable or even painful so the doctor should use a local anaesthetic cream. Chris describes how seven-year-old Abbey has regular IVs to combat infection:

'Once the line is in she has to have the antibiotics every eight hours – so I do it at 8 a.m. when she gets up, 4 p.m. when she comes home from school, and midnight while she is asleep. I have to flush out the line first then the antibiotic goes in very slowly, then I flush the line out again. To start with it took me an hour but now I can do it in 20–30 minutes. The worst bit is when they put the line in: she gets really distressed if it doesn't go in first or second time. Last time they gave her gas and air and it was brilliant: she kept popping up and saying "Let me look".'

A course of IVs usually lasts for 14 days and if a line is handled carefully then it will last for the whole course. If IVs are given very frequently it may become difficult to find a place to put the line. It is at this stage that children or adults are sometimes offered a 'totally implantable venous access device' or Port-A-Cath. A small device is put under the skin where it can stay for years, providing an easy way in for the IV antibiotics. Even six-year-olds have been known to manage very well with a Port-A-Cath. Home IVs and Port-A-Caths are brilliant for school-age children because they enable the children to carry on going to school – if they feel well enough – which reinforces the idea that they can live a normal life and helps to make sure they don't fall behind in their studies or miss out on seeing their friends.

Pancreatic enzymes – see below

Vitamins

Children with CF need to have extra vitamins in the form of drops or tablets every day. This is because many vitamins – particularly the fat-soluble A, D and E – are not absorbed very well from the food they eat.

DNase

DNase is an enzyme which breaks down the mucus produced in the airways, thins it out and makes it easier to cough up. It is inhaled using a nebulizer (see box below). You may hear or read about this, although it's unlikely a young child will be offered DNase because it is currently only licensed for children over five. What's more, very young children are less likely to have large amounts of mucus. In the United States, however, it is now being evaluated in young children. You may be offered it if your child seems to have particularly thick mucus which is causing problems, but it only seems to work in about one in five people and at the moment doctors can't predict who is likely to benefit from it.

Bronchodilators

These drugs are given to relax spasms in the bronchial tube which cause wheezing and shortness of breath, as in asthma. The drugs can be given with a nebulizer.

Nebulizers
A nebulizer is a machine which converts a drug into a fine mist which can be inhaled. Babies can use a mask which covers the nose and mouth. Once they get older, children can be taught to use a mouthpiece, taking a few deep breaths through the mouth to get the drug deep into the lungs. Using a nebulizer means the antibiotic gets straight to the place where it's needed, less is used and there is less risk of any toxic effects.

Drug side effects
All drugs have possible side effects, most of them very rare. Whenever your child is prescribed a different drug it is important to get all the information about side effects so that you know what to look for.

Diet

Children with CF need more calories than other children of the same age if they are to grow at a normal rate and build up resistance to infection. But just like other children they can be faddy eaters and even refuse whole meals – simply because they are children, and that's what children do from time to time. Most parents get cross, frustrated and concerned when their child refuses to eat or eats very little. But if your child has CF you are naturally going to be particularly concerned, especially if you see the weight start to drop. It is important not to let mealtimes become a battle or to show how concerned you are: even very young children can be incredibly good at picking up on your anxiety and may use refusal to eat to manipulate you. Karen has learnt to compromise in order to keep the peace with her four-year-old son:

'It's very difficult to get him to eat. Even though he's four now I feed one meal to him. Even if he only has a bite out of a sandwich at teatime, at least I know he's had one good meal. People say "Oh you're flapping" but lots of parents I know feed their children until they're eight or nine just to make sure they get something.'

And sometimes you just have to be patient, as Paula recalls:

'When she was younger Sally used to be very fussy about her food. She knew I worried and I think she used it as a tool to battle with. Now she's ten she seems to have outgrown that, although I do have to get on to her sometimes.'

In general, parents whose children refuse to eat at mealtimes are advised not to give snacks in between meals. The same principle doesn't apply when a child has CF, however. Even when a child with CF does eat meals she may well need high-calorie snacks like milkshakes in between times.

People with CF are advised to eat full cream milk, full fat margarine or butter, cream and full fat cheese. During a chest infection it is even more important to keep eating because your child needs more energy, but their appetite may seem to vanish. If they lose weight during an infection it can be hard to put it on again afterwards, as Glenda discovered:

'It's a myth that all children with CF have voracious appetites. They may have no appetite at all and children are difficult to feed at the best of times. If you've got a CF child with a poor appetite you've got double the anxiety. What do you do? You worry! There isn't any solution really: I just gave my daughter what she wanted.'

Other parents have found they have no problems whatsoever with getting their children to eat.

'We're lucky she has a good appetite. In fact she eats us out of house and home. I just let her eat as much as she likes.' (Judy, mother of Ellen aged seven)

'We've never had any problems getting him to eat – in fact, if anything, he's overweight now.' (Angela, mother of Peter aged 15)

Keeping up a good weight can also be important for your child's self image and to reinforce the point that they are in almost all respects just like anyone else.

You should expect to see a dietician on a fairly regular basis – perhaps twice a year or more often if you are having particular problems with your child's diet. Doctors today are very conscious of the fact that CF is not simply a chest condition: weight gain is vital and weight loss is serious. Children who get a high fat, high calorie diet can achieve average or near average height and have a better chance of surviving into adulthood. Weight gain is also dependent in part on getting enough pancreatic enzymes to control diarrhoea.

Enzymes

The digestive problems caused by CF are in large part due to the fact that the enzymes or digestive juices produced in the pancreas can't get through because of sticky mucus lining the passages. However, it is possible to replace most of the missing enzymes with a medicine called pancreatin which has to be taken before any food – even snacks.

Pancreatin comes in two main forms – capsules or powders. The capsule dissolves in the stomach releasing specially coated particles called enteric coated microspheres which are designed to resist stomach acid as they pass through on their way to the duodenum – the lower part of the gut – where they are thought to work best.

It is safe to give pancreatin in powder form to babies: you can mix it with a small amount of milk (formula or breast milk) or cooled boiled water and give it before a feed. Once your baby is taking solid food you can mix the powder with a spoonful of the puréed food you're about to give her. As with older children, it may take a while to get the dose of pancreatin right. If your baby tends to feed little and often it may not be necessary to give pancreatin before every single feed. Parents find their own ways of getting children to take the enzymes, as Karen discovered:

'They suggested we put the Creon [a brand name for pancreatin] in fruit purée but that was a bit sour for Robert so we put it in yoghurt. Now he's four he gets through 50–70 yoghurts a week – really high fat ones. He's just had four chocolate mousses before going to bed!'

If you're having problems finding a way to get your baby or child to take the enzymes it's important to get help sooner rather than later: dieticians who specialize in CF are likely to have met the problem in the past and should have lots of ideas for dealing with it.

Getting it right

Pancreatin sometimes has to be taken in what seem like alarming quantities. It is not unheard of, for example, for a ten-year-old child to be taking 70 tablets a day. Your doctors will advise you how much to give although it may take some time to get the dose right. As a general rule, if your child suffers from diarrhoea and smelly poo and doesn't grow well then she is probably not having enough pancreatin. If she is constipated and has a sore bottom she is probably getting too much. Tummy aches can be a problem in both cases so they aren't a very reliable indicator either way, although regular tummy aches may be a sign that the pancreatin dose needs changing.

If your child goes to school and is responsible for his or her own pancreatin it might be worth investigating how much he or she is actually taking. Some children are embarrassed about the number of tablets they have to take before school dinner and either hide or 'lose' them. Others simply forget, as Paula explains:

'Sally is very forgetful. Sometimes I know she forgets to take her enzymes before her dinner. Other times she'll take them at snack time and then forget to have her snack! I have to ask her about it every day.'

Vitamins and minerals

There is a risk that children with CF won't get enough zinc and the vitamins which are dissolved in fat – particularly vitamins A, D, E and K – because these trace elements aren't being absorbed properly in the intestine. Although they are only ever required in tiny amounts, vitamins and minerals have very important jobs to do. Zinc, for example, plays a part in growth and puberty so that stunted growth and delayed puberty are both associated with zinc deficiency (although puberty is much more likely to be delayed in adolescents with CF because of low weight). Zinc may also keep the thymus gland and the immune system healthy. However, when people with CF have been given zinc supplements the results have not been particularly astonishing: only occasionally have the supplements led to improved growth.

The CF clinic may recommend vitamin supplements for your child, but don't give any other supplements yourself: too much of a good thing can be harmful.

Salt

Because people with CF tend to produce a lot of salt in their sweat they may need to take in extra salt during hot weather. Look out for signs of lethargy and ask your doctor if your child needs salt tablets.

Feeding supplements

If you are finding it hard to get your child to eat enough your doctor and dietician may prescribe a dietary or feeding supplement such as Fortisip, Fortison, Ensure or Caloreen. These come as either liquids for drinking or as powders which you can add to drinks. You may also be offered high calorie tinned puddings or other fortified foods.

Breastfeeding a baby with CF

There is no reason why babies with CF shouldn't benefit from breastmilk in the same way as other babies, and it may be very important to you that you can give your baby all the positive health advantages of breastfeeding, including the transfer of your antibodies which can help protect against infections. Breastmilk also contains proteins which are more easily digested and fat which is more easily absorbed than the proteins and fats in formula milk. Breastfeeding can also help mothers to feel they are doing everything they possibly can for their babies. Even so, you may find you're under pressure to switch to formula milk if the baby doesn't gain weight. If this is the case it may be possible to go for mixed feeding – a combination of formula and breastmilk.

Because breastmilk is so easily digested, it is possible a fully breastfed baby might not need enzymes, but there are no guarantees. If breastfed babies don't gain weight this is an indication that they may need the enzymes. If you bottlefeed, your baby is almost certainly going to need enzymes before a feed.

The enzymes can be mixed with water or a little expressed milk or formula milk. You can give this on a spoon or from a special baby-feeding cup if you are breastfeeding and you don't want to use a bottle. Bottlefeeding requires a different sucking technique from your baby and in the early days using a bottle can confuse a baby who is still learning to feed from the breast.

If pancreatin comes into contact with the skin and isn't wiped away it can cause some soreness. As a result, if you are breastfeeding you may notice your nipples get sore. You can help prevent this by washing your breasts with water after each feed.

Physiotherapy

Along with diet, physiotherapy is the cornerstone of treatment for CF. Its role is to clear the thick mucus from your child's chest and has to be done daily, twice a day usually, from the time your child is diagnosed. The exact amount of physiotherapy and the technique to be used depends very much on how badly your child's lungs are affected, the age of the child and whether there is a chest infection at the time (longer and more frequent physio is needed to help clear the extra secretions that occur during an infection). So a session lasting 10–15 minutes might be enough normally, but this might increase to 45–60 minutes if your child has a very bad cough and is bringing up a lot of mucus. Once they are nine or ten many children will be able to do their own physio: until then you, your partner and other carers will have to take responsibility.

Physiotherapy involves assessing your child – looking to see if he is breathing noisily or more quickly than normal, for example, and feeling for rattles or crackles in his chest, and then constantly watching during the treatment to monitor the secretions and the way your child is responding to the physio.

The treatment itself involves draining secretions from different parts of the lung using chest 'clapping' – clapping a cupped hand onto the chest – and gentle shaking. This is done in a variety of positions so that all parts of the lung are cleared and so gravity can help bring the secretions up to be coughed out of the lungs. Your child doesn't have to spit out mucus: so long as the secretions are coughed out of the lungs they can be swallowed. Later on your child can be taught special breathing techniques which can also help to relax the airways and clear secretions.

It is not surprising if this sounds daunting – the reliance on a routine, the time involved and the skills you're going to need. As with all skills, it is very unlikely you'll 'get it right' first time, and the physiotherapists involved in teaching the techniques should give you lots of encouragement and opportunities to practise. Even when you've been doing the physio for a while it makes sense to let the physiotherapist watch you doing it from time to time, to check your child is getting the most out of each session and because a child's needs change as they get older and are able to get more involved in the treatment. The Cystic Fibrosis Trust* produces a booklet called *The physical treatment of cystic fibrosis*, which gives a lot of detail about the different physiotherapy techniques.

Some parents have found it helps to turn physio into a game, which babies and young children seem to enjoy. It may also help to see it as a very special, close and physical time you can spend with your child. It's a good idea if several people involved with your child can learn how to do the physio – so it doesn't all fall to one person who may feel burdened or may simply be ill or unavailable on occasions. Karen recalls how she felt when she first needed to do baby Robert's physio:

'I felt very nervous to start with, doing it on a baby. So I asked someone from the support group to come and show me because she'd done it on a baby herself. It's actually really easy with a baby: we'd do it for half an hour in the evening and he'd just fall asleep.'

Foam wedges and frames
While your child is still a baby, physio can be done while she lays on your lap. When she gets older you'll need a foam wedge and then a specially designed physio bed which tips to allow drainage from different parts of the lungs. Ask your physiotherapist for details of equipment suppliers or ask around to see if anyone has any second-hand equipment their children have outgrown.

But physiotherapy needn't be a chore. As Judy recalls:

'It's weird because we were doing physio instinctively for Ellen's cough, even before she was actually diagnosed with CF. So we just carried on and she's never found it distressing. In fact, as a baby and toddler she used to fall asleep while we were doing it. I think she found it comforting. She's never brought up a load of sputum because her chest is actually very clear, so it's more of a comfort thing.'

The situation can change as your child gets older, of course, not only because you may need to use different techniques and equipment (see box above), but because toddlers tend to be more stroppy than babies and seven-year-olds can answer back! Karen and Glenda describe how they reached a compromise with their young children:

'Once Robert was one or two, physio was the last thing he wanted: he'd be running around and it was really difficult to pin him down. Now we just do it in the evening for 20 or 30 minutes after a bath when he's relaxed. We only do it in the morning if he's unwell.'

'I used to go into school during the lunch hour to give my daughter physio but it used to make her really miserable, so in the end I gave up and we compromised on two sessions a day, night and morning. You've got to balance quality of life and longevity.'

Occasionally a real battle can develop, however, and you may need to walk away from the situation or get someone else involved just to diffuse the tension, as Paula describes:

'I do find the physio very time-consuming. Sally's ten now and she really hates it. She's not too bad about doing her breathing exercises, but then she starts fidgeting and I'm just standing there waiting. I wait for ten minutes and then I walk away. Then she shouts out "You're killing me. I'm going to die." I know she's just using it as a guilt thing but I can't win whatever I do. It's like she's using it as a control thing to get my attention. We have to do it as soon as she gets up in the morning and she's really grumpy then. It's better at night when I go off to work and her stepfather does it. She's okay with him.'

Exercise

Not only is regular exercise possible for people with CF, it's very important:

- Fitter people feel less breathless because muscles become more efficient at using the available oxygen.
- Exercise slows the deterioration of lung function.
- It helps clear sputum out of the lungs and so may reduce the number of infections.
- Exercise can increase muscle bulk which can be useful if you are very thin.
- It makes you feel good since it produces substances called endorphins which are your body's natural equivalent of pain-killing happy pills.
- It reinforces the truth that people with CF can lead a 'normal' life, doing 'normal' things and mixing with 'normal' people.
- Moderate exercise enhances your ability to fight infections.

On the other hand, people with CF should avoid excessive exercise which can go the opposite way and decrease immunity. But there is no reason why your toddler shouldn't go to 'Tumbletots', have a trampet in the playroom and a climbing frame in the garden, or why your school-age child shouldn't cycle in the park and take part in PE, swimming and playground games such as football and skipping. Regular physical activity is particularly important for girls who tend to have less well-developed muscles. Going to a gym from an early age may encourage both girls and boys to see regular exercise as part of everyday life. Paula has found that there's just about nothing Sally isn't able to tackle:

'She does horse riding, ballet and swimming. When I tell mothers of CF babies, they're amazed, but she's really very fit. There's no way you'd know she'd got CF, to look at her.'

27

Chris says that her daughter Abbey wants to have a go at everything:

> 'And she can – except I don't let her play outside in damp and cold weather. She does tend to cough a lot when she's exercising or when she goes from the cold to the warm, and when she's tired her breathing is fast and erratic, but mostly she keeps up and does very well.'

The environment

Anybody with lung problems should avoid smoking, smokers and passive smoking of any kind because of the damage it can do to the lungs. If your child has CF it's important to avoid smokers and smoky atmospheres as much as possible. If you, your partner or any regular visitors to the house smoke, it's vital you discuss this with your child's doctor and get help in giving up.

Once children are socializing with other children it will be impossible to protect them from picking up infections from time to time. Obviously it makes sense to keep them away from people with streaming colds and hacking coughs but otherwise there's very little point in isolating them from their playmates. There will always be these difficult decisions to make – balancing your child's need for a normal life with your desire to protect. Different parents will take a different approach and you will need to work out what's right for you and your child.

Going to school

There is usually no reason at all why children with CF shouldn't go to the ordinary, local school. But it makes sense to talk to the staff at the school and make sure they understand what CF is and what implications it has. In particular it is worth discussing:

- Coughing: children with CF must be allowed to cough as often and as loudly as they need to, although this is potentially disruptive in the classroom. Teachers will need to find a way of explaining this to the rest of the class who may try to imitate the coughing for a laugh or to be disruptive.
- Taking pancreatin: since the enzymes need to be taken before any food is eaten – whether at break time or dinner time, a teacher may need to look after the tablets and give them out at the appropriate time. But teachers aren't obliged to supervise or give medicines, and each school will have its own policy about medicines.

- School meals: the average school meal probably won't provide enough fat, protein and carbohydrate for a child with CF. You could discuss with the school whether it is possible for your child to have larger portions, extra bread or a top-up from home, such as a high-energy drink as well as a big snack at break time.
- PE: children with CF can benefit enormously from exercise (see above) but the teachers must be on the look-out for signs of strain such as wheezing.
- Catching-up work: children with CF sometimes miss school for weeks at a time if they have a bad infection. It helps a lot if the class teacher can provide catching-up work so that the child doesn't fall behind.
- Physio during the day: if this is necessary, and you have a good relationship with the school, you may be able to come in and take your child to a quiet room for half an hour or so. If one of the teachers is able to learn how to do the physio this means your child will be able to go on school trips.
- Siblings at school: if you have other children at school it's important their class teachers know what is happening in case these children react to what is going on at home (see chapter 5).

Under the 1993 Education Act schools have a responsibility for identifying any special needs children may have. The Special Educational Needs co-ordinator (often referred to as the Special Needs teacher) will probably take the lead in working out with you what your child needs – if anything – in the way of extra help. Having a good relationship with this teacher, and with your child's class teacher, will help enormously: both you and your child are likely to be more relaxed about school if you know you can go in and chat about things as they crop up.

If you have any problems in dealing with your child's school, you can get help from the Cystic Fibrosis Trust* Family and Adult Support Services (FASS) department. For example, if teachers seem concerned, particularly about administering or supervising medicines, your local FASS worker may be able to go with you to the school to reassure them or may be able to refer them to other teachers who have taken on this responsibility. Most parents find they have a good relationship with the school and very few problems:

'When he started at school the health visitor and the physio came to the school to have a chat to the teachers. At the moment he doesn't need to have physio at school but if he ever does the hospital physio said she'd come in and show them how to do it. He loves school but he's not very happy with having school dinners because he's used to me giving him his food. He's a bit lazy – a typical boy really. So I just give him a yoghurt to take in and the teacher gives him his Creon [a brand name for pancreatin] to put on the top. The other kids don't ask about the Creon – they just want his yoghurts!' (Karen, mother of Robert aged four)

'We've never had any problems with the school. They've always made her feel very special and when there was the Blue Peter appeal for cystic fibrosis she spoke in assembly. At dinner time the dinner ladies give her the little capsules she has to have with food. Sometimes her friends ask why she has to take so many medicines and I just say it's because her belly doesn't work. She's never been one to hide it and I think the other kids are just inquisitive.' (Judy, mother of Ellen aged seven)

'We told the school and his close friends and I did have to go in sometimes to do physio. He's never particularly wanted to hide it and if the kids ask about his enzymes he says it's because he can't digest food: he doesn't mention CF – they wouldn't understand.' (Angela, mother of Peter aged 15)

'The school had never had someone with CF before and I think they were quite frightened really, but I didn't want them to wrap her in cotton wool. I'm very matter of fact about it and she wants to have a go at everything. The school have been brilliant: the Special Needs teacher handles her Creon and antibiotics and when she misses a week they send home work for her to do here.' (Chris, mother of Abbey aged seven)

Unfortunately, some schools are less than helpful, as Paula discovered when she moved house:

'The first school Sally went to was very good about it, but the next one wasn't. They refused to help her take her tablets, they wanted her to do it. They just didn't want the responsibility and no one would take it on. They said "It's her disease, she should do it", which I thought was a bit much since she was only eight at the time and she is very forgetful. All we wanted was someone to remind her and supervise. Fortunately the dinner ladies are quite good and the secretary agreed to help with her antibiotics at break time. But she doesn't like people staring at her.'

It's very important to make sure that all the teachers who will be involved with your child have a good understanding of the condition and how much it means to children with CF that they are treated normally. Tracey, who is now 22, says she remembers going to school and one of the teachers saying 'You'll rattle if you eat all those tablets':

'It really put me off taking them in public for ages, and even now I don't like it. I think I was sort of scarred by what she said.'

Later on, if your child does need extra help at school, it may be important to get your child statemented. A statement or 'statutory statement' comes from the local education authority (LEA). It's basically a statement of your child's special educational needs which the LEA then monitors and reviews. Whether or not children with CF need statementing when they start school, it may help to meet the people involved so you understand the process. Angela explains what statementing means for her 15-year-old son Peter:

'Basically it means that someone is supposed to find out what he's missed when he can't go to school because he's ill. They've also organized these catch-up periods for him – so he's dropped languages altogether and uses the time to catch up with his other work then.'

A similar system operates in Scotland where it may be possible for a 'record of needs' to be opened for your child. This is only likely to be done if there are significant difficulties with learning as well as physical difficulties.

Being normal

Above all else, most children with CF want to be treated as normally as possible. Glenda's experience with her daughter Julie reinforces that:

'If you asked my daughter when was her worst time she'd say when she was seven or eight because she was put on steroids for a time and her face blew up like a munchkin. She said "I'd rather die than look like that again". It's so important to her to be normal, to be integrating with others on a normal level.'

Financial help

It may be possible to claim benefits such as Disability Living Allowance (DLA) if your child has CF. DLA is a benefit for people under 65 who need help with personal care. Staff at the Cystic Fibrosis Trust* Family and Adult Support Services department are trained to help you complete the application form and can give you up-to-date advice related to your individual circumstances.

Questions and answers

Should I have my child immunized?
Yes. Routine immunizations are recommended since children with CF are particularly at risk from common childhood diseases, especially those which may affect the lungs. The vaccinations are as safe for children with CF as for other children, so long as you take the usual precautions: they should not be given while your child has a chest infection, for example. Once babies are six months old they should also have a flu jab each year at the beginning of winter.

Do we have to tell the school that our child has CF?
No, you're not obliged to do this by law. Some parents just want their child to be treated like everyone else, and that's fair enough. But you need to think through what the teachers and other pupils might say when your child is taking enzymes before food or when your child coughs a lot in class, for example. Before making your decision not to say anything it would be worth talking it through with other parents. Your local Family and Adult Support Services worker can put you in touch with some.

'If I was asked to give advice to parents whose child has just been diagnosed with CF I'd like them to meet me and say, "Oh good, she looks so well." You've got every reason to be positive. There will be a cure.' (Tracey, aged 22)

3

Getting good care

'You start off and you think the care's wonderful but as you know a bit more you see lapses. You have to ask more questions and demand more.'

Specialist care

Most consultant paediatricians working in ordinary local hospitals will have at most 20 patients with CF. Because they are dealing with such a wide range of conditions these doctors rarely have the time to keep up to date with the very latest research on CF and its treatment. Neither do local hospitals have the range of specialist CF staff who make up the multidisciplinary teams working out of the specialist centres. These teams include not only doctors but nurses, social workers, physiotherapists, dieticians and psychologists, all with a special interest and training in cystic fibrosis.

But some people have a lot of trouble getting referred to a specialist centre. As one of the CF Trust* Family and Adult Support Services (FASS) workers comments:

'There is a huge variation in care among non-specialist clinics, and paediatricians working out of local hospitals are often loath to let patients go, perhaps because of their frail egos. You can ask your GP for a referral, but GPs often don't know a lot about it so they just refer people back to the local paediatrician. But people with CF need holistic care, not just medical care.'

She recommends people to ask their GPs if they can see a CF specialist as a one-off, just to reassure themselves they understand everything. Then, she often finds, the specialist centre takes them on. It is clearly important to know the system and the local personalities involved, and this is where FASS workers are invaluable. Even if you are happy with the care you are getting, it is worth chatting to your local FASS worker to see if you are missing out on something. If you contact the CF Trust* you will be given the name and phone number of a local support worker.

Although Paula is happy with the care her daughter is getting at the local hospital she is aware that local people who want to transfer to the specialist centre about 40 miles away from her do have problems:

'I don't think they like you leaving because they lose money. You really have to push for it.'

Chris has no regrets about her decision to get her daughter's case transferred to a specialist centre, even though it means a 25-mile journey for her three-monthly appointments and usually one or two visits in between:

'I wasn't very happy with the local hospital at all. Abbey was put on mixed wards where children had all sorts of different conditions, and the care wasn't very good. Once they were six hours late giving her antibiotics and she often had Creon [a brand name for pancreatin] after she'd had her food because they'd forgotten it. She got better care at home than she got there. I did approach the consultant at the hospital and told him I wasn't very happy and I spoke to some other mums whose children were at the specialist centre, then I told my GP who referred us to the centre where we've been ever since. They're brilliant: they're on call 24 hours a day and they never tell me I'm fussing when I bring her in.'

Chris agrees, though, that you need to fight for what you want sometimes, or be prepared to do some research of your own. She recalls how she disagreed with the way the hospital were refusing to sedate Abbey when they tried time after time to insert a line for her IVs:

'In the end they were holding her down and you don't treat animals like that. They said they wouldn't sedate her because of the damage it might do to her lungs but I felt they should have stopped trying after the third time. Afterwards I contacted the next nearest specialist centre and they told me they would have put a Port-A-Cath in. So when we went back I insisted they do something and last time they gave her gas and air and it was brilliant.'

If you're unhappy with the way something is being done then it's important to make a stand: not only for the sake of your child's health but also so you know you are doing all you can. Karen found that she had to devise her own system for improving the care her son got from the hospital:

'He'd have a cough swab done, but by the time we found out he was growing something four weeks would have gone by – and it was all because of poor communication. When it had happened a couple of times, and he'd been quite poorly in between, I thought "My son's health comes first", so a week after the cough swab I ring the consultant's secretary and she tells our GP the result. You've got to be on the ball.'

Even if you are getting good treatment at your local hospital it is worth checking out what help might be available from specialists. David recalls how they were introduced to the idea of shared care from the local and specialist hospitals about five years after his son Andrew was diagnosed:

'We were very happy with the care we were getting at the local hospital but when Andrew was seven or eight the paediatrician said she wanted to get other people involved. We weren't that keen but we went to see a specialist and from then on had shared care with the specialist centre and the local hospital. That first time we were at the specialist centre for two and a quarter hours but I don't think we wasted a minute. Even when we were in the waiting room we could talk to other families. When we did see the consultant, he said "You tell me about his condition", and that was his philosophy – it was as if he was saying "I may be the specialist, but you're the experts", and that attitude helps to develop a good relationship. We always felt he was working with us. It was good to get into a wider net of people with CF and I suppose the general level of treatment improved, but the local hospital was excellent. We had no complaints.'

Some people find it helps to meet up with other CF families going to the specialist clinic at the same time. On the other hand, it can be distressing to see other people who are now seriously ill, and there are concerns about the possibility of cross-infection (see chapter 6).

Local care may also be hindered by budgetary problems. It is not unheard of for a child with CF to be refused DNase or nebulized antibiotics because of the cost to the GP (DNase currently costs around £8,000 per patient per year).

If care is shared between a local hospital and a specialist centre then it is normal to have routine appointments every three months, with an annual check-up at the specialist centre. This annual check-up is recommended by experts as something all people with CF should have.

Medical notes are often held in both places, so that you can go straight to the specialist centre if necessary.

Routine clinic visits

These visits usually include:

- height and weight measurements;
- lung function test (whether or not there is an infection);
- discussion with the paediatrician;
- questions about coughing, wheezing, sputum, appetite, bowel habits and other symptoms;
- annual chest X-ray.

Other tests might include:

- Chest scans: radioactive substances are injected or inhaled into the body. These safe substances get into the lungs and the scan can show if there are parts of the lungs getting too little air or blood. Scans provide a more detailed picture than a chest X-ray.
- Bronchodilator test: if the lung function test suggests there may be a bronchospasm (a tightening of the airways) then the test may be repeated after your child has been given a bronchodilator drug to relax the bronchial tubes. If the lung function is improved then the drug is prescribed so it can be taken on a regular basis.

Extra visits

Specialist centres tend to have a 24-hour open-door policy, which means you are able to take your child there straightaway if you feel something is wrong. For Chris, this is a lifeline:

'It's definitely the most scary part – thinking when do I take her to the hospital? Should you leave it or should you go? I tend to take her straightaway because I don't want her lungs to get damaged – and nine times out of ten I'm right. The staff are great when you do go in.'

The CF Trust is currently discussing the possibility of accrediting clinics. This means that in the future clinics will have a model of good practice and standards to aim for.

Seeing the psychologist

Initially you might wonder what help a psychologist can offer – especially if your child is very young, but psychologists can help with a wide range of issues. In particular they are there to help you have a greater understanding of your child's behaviour and how to deal with certain situations. Angela went to see the psychologist on her own because she was concerned about how to broach certain subjects with her 15-year-old son Peter:

'She was brilliant and very very understanding. I wanted to know how to tell him about not being able to have children and she was really helpful. We also went to see her when he was having sleeping problems.'

Paula found the psychologist she saw was able to help explain what was going on with her daughter Sally who seemed to be fighting her all the time:

'She explained how Sally is very dominant and how she was using situations to control me. We talked about how I could try to get control back and what I could do. It was good to have someone to talk to who could understand and see what was happening.'

If you are going to a specialist centre then you have this kind of back-up resource available. But in many cases it will be up to you to take the first step and make use of it.

Getting the most out of your GP

It varies how much GPs get involved in the care of patients with CF. Because CF is a long-term condition involving regular routine hospital appointments, then it may not be necessary to involve the GP at all. As Judy explains:

'I always go straight to the hospital if I need anything really, unless it's just a cough in which case I'll ask the GP if we can up her antibiotics.'

If you want your GP to be more involved then:

- choose a GP who acknowledges their need to refer, who allows the family to be the experts and who has a policy of sharing information and care;
- build up a relationship by keeping in touch;
- have realistic expectations – GPs aren't CF specialists;
- swap information;
- make clear arrangements about repeat prescriptions;
- understand the night and weekend on-call arrangements.

4

Coping as individuals and as a couple

'They said she's got cystic fibrosis and I didn't even know what it was.
I just went into a daze and kept thinking over and over this isn't
happening, this isn't happening. My husband's not like me. He was
asking loads of questions straightaway: what does it mean? how long
will she live? But I just ran out of the room. I couldn't take it.'

Most people who have got a child with CF describe how deeply shocked
they were when they were first given the diagnosis. Whether or not you
know much about CF at that stage, it seems frightening, partly perhaps
because it's a condition, not a bug which can be dealt with quickly. It's
something which will go on being there. After the initial shock, however,
feelings vary. Many people speak of the relief they felt that at last they
could start doing something positive to help their child who had been so
ill. Others say they became absorbed in the practical detail of coping – so
much so that their emotions were put on a back burner for a while. As one
mother commented:

'The practical side of it isn't so much a problem – the drugs and the
diet. It's the emotional side, accepting what's happened, that takes
time.'

And as one father remarks:

'I don't know to what extent the implications sank in at the time.
You've got a situation and you've got to get on with it.'

You may still be at this point and this chapter may represent the first
chance you've had to really examine your feelings about CF. If so, take
your time to really think, because people have very different emotional
reactions. Some of the things you'll read you can just dismiss because
they don't apply to you – they simply won't reflect the way you are
feeling. Others may strike a chord.

The grieving process

The dictionary definition of grief is 'deep sorrow'. Grieving is not the
same as mourning, although it can be caused by loss, and in some ways
finding out your child has CF can represent a loss – the loss of the healthy

child you'd been expecting. So the grieving process is relevant to the way you cope with having a CF child.

It has long been recognized that grieving involves several stages. These have been described as:

- denial;
- confusion or anger;
- bargaining (with God, for example);
- depression;
- acceptance.

This is not to say that everyone goes through each clearly defined stage in this exact order. In reality there is a lot of blurring as your feelings naturally change from day to day. But in general there is a pattern, involving:

- immediate reaction: you're in shock and may even deny what is happening;
- developing awareness: sometimes you feel guilty or angry, other times you feel despondent or apathetic;
- full realization: you may feel depressed, empty or despairing;
- resolution: you accept the diagnosis and start to reorganize your life around it.

Shock can have different effects on people. Some people are simply frozen: life seems to go on around them but it has no meaning for them as they walk around in a daze with the thinking part of their brain not really switched on. Others go into overdrive as they dash around hyperactively, but again not really thinking or allowing themselves an opportunity to feel very much.

Some people start off with a tremendous feeling of relief as soon as they get the diagnosis. This may be particularly true if your child has been very ill, in and out of hospital and not gaining weight. It can be a relief to have a diagnosis at last, even though it is a serious one. You may always have believed there was something wrong and feel vindicated at last. In this case the shock may come later when the reality of the diagnosis sinks in. Getting the diagnosis is, after all, only the beginning. As one Family and Adult Support Services (FASS) worker whose daughter has CF explained:

'The way you feel changes. To start with you're in denial and then you start frantically searching for a cure. You feel you've got to do something positive to help.'

Perhaps reading this book is, for you, part of the grieving process. Sometimes gathering information is what psychologists call a 'displacement activity' – something we do to stop ourselves focusing on the real issue. There's nothing wrong with that, since finding out more can help you cope on a practical level, but it's important to acknowledge what you are doing and why. As one mother commented:

'People these days are very good about getting information. You can know all the facts but you still have to accept it. Nobody can do that bit for you.'

Why me?

If you never have this thought then you're in the minority. Being told that your child has a life-threatening condition is bound to rock your world and your sense of justice. If you have a religious faith then that too may be rocked or even shattered if you feel you have been let down by your God.

The element of chance involved in CF seems so cruel: it was a one-in-625 chance that both you and your partner would carry the CF gene, and then a one-in-four chance that your child would have it. A tiny one-in-2,500 chance – and your baby was the one.

There's very little which can be said to take away this feeling of injustice. Some people take comfort from the idea that their child is special and – if they have a faith – believe they have been chosen by God to look after this very special person. Others find this idea abhorrent. Some people are able to take a pragmatic view that at least they know the score, and they can make every day count from now on. And the truth is, that you aren't the only one: every year about 250 couples find themselves in exactly your position. Hundreds of others discover that their babies are suffering from leukaemia, heart problems or congenital abnormalities. That doesn't mean you should just snap out of it and start counting your blessings. Of course not. But it does show you that despite all the great advances in medical science, these things do happen and you aren't on your own in having to come to terms with the disappointment, the anger, the agony and the bitterness. People reach this point at different times, as Karen, mother of four-year-old Robert, discovered:

'Every day my husband thinks about our son and his condition and when he goes out he's always thinking "Why couldn't it have been you,

41

or you?" He hasn't come to terms with it 100 per cent and he's always thinking about it. But me, I think you've got to look on the bright side. Life's lovely at the moment.'

David, the father of a grown-up son with CF, finds it really does help him to put CF in a wider perspective:

'I was talking to the mother of a haemophiliac the other day and at the end of the conversation we both said, at the same time, "I don't know how you cope". It's good to be reminded there's always someone somewhere who's worse off.'

Guilt

Feeling guilty because you have 'given' your child CF is both rational and irrational at the same time. Rational because it's a fact that your genes and those of your partner have caused the condition. Irrational because there was no intention to pass on CF, no carelessness on your part, and no selfishness involved:

'When she cries I say "If I could have CF instead of you I would, but I can't".' (Judy, mother of Ellen aged seven)

'There's always lots of guilt around and you find you blame each other. That's crazy of course, but such situations are crazy.' (Barbara, grandmother of Chris, an adult with CF)

Mandy was diagnosed as having CF when she was 18 so she is able to recall her parents' reaction to the news:

'When we found out I had CF my parents were very shocked. Dad kept saying over and over that he didn't know there was anything wrong. I was just about to leave home at the time so I wasn't there to see how they coped, but I know they came to terms with it very slowly. We all had to convince ourselves that it was mild, but it was a long slow process. I think they felt very guilty.'

There may perhaps be times when you'll wish you could turn back the clock – and then feel immediately guilt-stricken for having that thought. But there will be many, many other times when your child gives you so much joy and delight that you have no regrets.

Guilt is an extremely destructive emotion, particularly if you keep it inside and never talk about it. Telling your partner how you feel – and probably finding he or she shares the same emotion – will help, but at some point you may have consciously to put the guilt on one side so you can get on with living and enjoying watching your child grow up. As one grandmother said:

'I felt some guilt too, but having seen my daughter-in-law so devastated by it I realized how pointless it was. It's like jealousy – a completely hopeless emotion. It's just chance, after all.'

Individuals and couples

Reactions to bereavement, although they usually follow the pattern outlined above, are highly individual and people vary in the extent to which they grieve publicly. Many people present one face to the world and quite another behind closed doors, or when they are alone. The obvious implication of this is that you and your partner may grieve in completely different ways and you may each have an impact on the other's grieving. So, for example, if one partner grieves very openly the other may feel the need to be strong and practical in public, shutting away the grief and later feeling bitter that the other partner wasn't supportive. Or one may appear cold and distanced from events to the extent that the other partner feels the need to compensate by demonstrating grief – again with repercussions later.

This needn't be the case, of course. Your relationship may be such that you share your feelings openly and support each other. Many couples do find that a crisis of some kind brings them together. Others find the opposite is true. If you feel that you can't get through to your partner or that things are just 'going wrong' somehow then it may be worth spending some time thinking what could be behind what is happening. The possible responses outlined below may ring some bells.

- *Opting out.* In reality this is more likely to be a reaction from the father, particularly if he is the major bread-winner. If he isn't around much during the day he won't be able to take an active part in physiotherapy, giving pancreatin or coping with routine clinic visits. Distancing himself may be his way of 'coping' with feelings of guilt, anger, frustration and bitter disappointment. He may even take on more work responsibilities (perhaps supposedly or in reality to make up for a loss of income if his partner decides not to return to work) – responsibilities which keep him away from the home for longer periods. In this way he can easily lose touch with his child and the reality of living with CF. He may even become dismissive of the effort involved – because he simply has no idea. As one mother said: 'Life with CF is so busy and men can feel left out of it. I think it's really important to at least take turns at physio.'

- *Depression and exhaustion.* The commitment and responsibility associated with caring for a child with CF can be physically demanding and emotionally draining. It's easy to become depressed and over-tired if you're the one doing most of the work and most of the worrying.
- *Denial.* One parent may deny the seriousness of the illness or the validity of the diagnosis. As one FASS worker explained: 'I know one couple who've split up because the partner just couldn't accept there was anything wrong because their child looks so normal. It's so bad that even now when she goes to stay with her dad he won't give her any treatment. People like this need a lot of help: for some reason they just can't accept something has gone wrong in their lives.'
- *Anger.* You may feel angry towards your partner if he or she always belittled or shrugged off your attempts to find out what was wrong with your child. Or you may feel angry if you hadn't wanted this child as much as your partner.
- *Guilt.* Most parents of CF children share this feeling that they are responsible for passing on the genes that caused this condition. Some partners may feel additional guilt if they didn't take their partner's concerns about the child's illness seriously. Someone who is opting out of responsibility may also be feeling very guilty but unable to get involved for some reason.
- *Exclusion.* Sometimes one parent (often the mother) can be overprotective towards the child, leaving the other out in the cold. This exclusion can sometimes precede opting out (see above). If one of you quickly becomes an 'expert' in CF the other may feel belittled, unwanted or clumsy when trying to help – with the result that they stop trying.
- *Failure.* Sometimes people feel they have 'failed' to produce a healthy child and that therefore they are less than a whole man or woman. It can be extremely difficult to admit to these feelings of failure and shame, and very difficult to talk about them to your partner. Instead you may become either very insecure and introverted or very aggressive. Sometimes it may be enough to admit the feelings to yourself and acknowledge how irrational they are (logic tells you that three times out of four your child would not have had CF).

Staying together

If any of the situations above apply to you, then you may decide you need to act now to save your relationship from deteriorating to one in which you function side by side but share very little of your real feelings. Sometimes all you may need is the chance to spend some time alone together. In the early days you are bound to be anxious about leaving your child with anyone else, but as time goes on and your child's needs become clearer it should be possible to find a mature babysitter for the evening or get a grandparent to step in at the weekend. All new parents have this need to rediscover their relationship each time a baby is born because the baby's needs upset the balance within the house. The same is true when CF is diagnosed.

Sometimes, though, even a regular night out isn't going to be enough. Other suggestions for action include:

- Talk about how you feel – with someone else there if necessary, perhaps a counsellor from Relate*, a FASS worker, or a social worker from the hospital. People who are trained listeners and counsellors can help you to talk to each other in a positive way which doesn't end in mud-slinging and recriminations. For example, they may get you to use a technique which involves 'owning' your own feelings. So instead of saying 'You never take any interest in what has gone on during the day', you could say 'I feel hurt when you don't seem to take an interest . . .'. People who have had this kind of counselling often say how helpful it was at clearing the air.
- Swap roles for a day or a week, or even permanently.
- Find other ways of being involved. If you or your partner can't be at home involved in the day-to-day care of your child then there are other ways of being involved and showing your commitment to the family. Gathering information (from books or the Internet), attending local support group meetings, or taking time off to attend hospital visits could help. Later on you might want to help with fundraising.
- Focus on what's normal about your child – which is everything except CF. Don't exclude yourselves from other couples with children the same age on the grounds that they can't understand. It's true, they can't. But you have heaps in common with them simply because you are parents and learning as you go along how to deal with your child. Later on your child will thank you for reinforcing the normality of life.
- Join a local support group where you have a chance to meet other couples who are coping with some of the same feelings as you. After meetings you can discuss with your partner what you have seen and

heard, and that may give you an opportunity to tell each other what you are thinking and feeling.

There's no doubt that couples cope in different ways: some stay together apparently from force of habit, although love is lost somewhere along the line. Others pick up the pieces and get on with life, accepting joint responsibility for making the relationship work. Some build their lives around CF; others just make it fit in:

'We say we're going through a rocky patch, but looking back it all started when we found out she'd got CF. We don't blame each other, but it puts such a strain on your relationship. Suddenly we became a team, not a couple. We're a team working for CF and it takes up a lot of our time – fundraising, meetings and everything else. It's around all the time.' (Judy, mother of Ellen aged seven)

'You can't help thinking what if. What if we'd never met? What if we hadn't got married? What if we'd stopped after two children? In the end, though, you look at the children and think I wouldn't swap them for the world.' (Mary, mother of Suzy aged four)

'My husband helped all the way. It was just having someone to talk to really. He can't completely understand what it's like for me, but I don't get down very often. When I do, I ring up a friend and we talk things through. I think we've coped really well as a family. We all get on well and we've pulled together. But there is a lot of stress. I feel as if I'm with it all day. I can't go out to work, even now he's 15, because he has long times off school.' (Angela, mother of Peter aged 15)

'To start with your whole evening was taken up with it and I suppose it did hold us back – stop us from going out in the past, but not now. It could take over your whole life if you let it.' (Karen, mother of Robert aged four)

'I think it's made us closer. It's really important to work together and it made us more determined than ever for our children. We're a really close family.' (Susan, mother of Peter and John, adults with CF)

'You build your life around a regime of physio and hospitals. By the time you've got time for each other you've forgotten what it's like. But to us, this is normal. Yes there are strains, but a lot of couples have strained marriages where there are no big problems.' (Margaret, mother of Andrew, an adult with CF)

It is important to remember that both you and your partner have needs too. Yes, CF is very demanding, even overwhelming, but if you ignore or suppress your own needs you are asking for trouble in the long run. Above all else, many of us need to feel loved and nurtured. Although sex isn't by any means the only way to express your love and caring for your partner, lack of it is often one reason why relationships fall apart. Sex is an act full of meaning: for men it can restore confidence, for women it can provide reassurance. Unfortunately, when a couple's sex life stops – and it's hardly surprising if the effort involved in coping with CF were to take over everything in the first few months – it takes great effort for either partner to broach the subject and get it started again. Sex somehow becomes awkward.

If this happens to you and your partner, you aren't alone. A recent survey of new parents found that it's not unheard of for couples not to have sex for up to two years or more after a baby is born, and only half of all couples say they have sex as frequently after having a baby. Children, it has been said, are the most effective contraceptive ever invented.

There is no single solution to a lack of sex: maybe your love life will never be quite the same again, but that doesn't mean it can't be good. (The same survey found many people commented spontaneously that although quantity had gone down, quality had gone up!) The first step is – as always – to talk to your partner about how you feel. It's much easier to write or read that than it is to do it, of course, although you may well find your partner is only too ready to talk because he or she has been thinking about exactly the same thing. One idea is to spend some time on your own remembering all the good times you have had together, and focusing on the things you have always valued about your partner and your relationship. Then – while you're feeling romantic and caring, rather than bitter and depressed – tell your partner how you feel: how much you miss being close or just spending time together.

If it's really impossible to get your partner talking – or if every discussion ends in disagreement or stalemate – then you could try seeing a sex therapist or Relate* counsellor who specializes in sex therapy. The Association of Sexual and Marital Therapists* will have lists of therapists working in your area. Although this kind of thing sounds really difficult, embarrassing or heavy, and is often the subject of sitcom antics, it needn't be like that. If you don't find the therapist sympathetic then you can always stop after one session. If your partner won't go with you then the therapist may be prepared to see you on your own (check first, though). People who have gone for sex therapy often find it is incredibly useful in helping them to work out why things have been going wrong and – importantly – to get them started again, enjoying sex as they did in the past. Wouldn't that be worth a bit of initial embarrassment?

Splitting up

One in three marriages ends within ten years. That fact alone suggests that marriage – or a long-term relationship – requires great effort and commitment from both partners. When a child is born with a life-threatening condition, the additional strain and the potential for disagreement and friction places a tremendous strain on relationships. Many end as a result. One mother whose daughter has CF explains how her first marriage ended under the strain of the diagnosis:

'She was diagnosed when she was three months old and I was in despair. My husband got very stressed by it all and couldn't cope with the fact that I gave all my attention to the baby. He hadn't really wanted children very much anyway so he left and we got divorced. He didn't really want to see her – he wouldn't see her unless I was able to go as well, but he was really just using the visits to talk to me. It wasn't until she was about two or three that he could cope. I did feel resentful at the time that he left it all to me, but later I could see why it happened: I was so bound up with it that I couldn't do anything else.'

Chris recalls how her marriage ended in fairly similar circumstances:

'He left us when Abbey was 18 months old. He'd never been able to handle the fact that she had CF. He'd had two children from his previous marriage and he kept saying he had healthy children. I don't know if it's ego or pride or what but he couldn't handle the fact that he was carrying a bad gene. He never got close to Abbey. He never cuddled her, and he always held her away from him as if she had something catching. And he resented me putting my efforts into looking after her. If I'm honest and put my hand on my heart I have to say I did neglect him – but he wasn't supportive. He gave me nothing. If he could have been there for me and waited it would have come back and been all right eventually. But he wouldn't get involved. He never visited her in hospital unless I took him and he never bought her anything. He just went out drinking all the time. He just buried his head in the sand and didn't want the responsibility.'

If you feel your relationship with your partner is threatened then it makes sense to get help – for example, from Relate* or Marriage Care*. Counsellors who specialize in relationships often say that their aim is not so much to help people to stay together as to help people to understand what is happening, so that, if they do decide to split up, at least they both understand why.

Having said that, once you are able to understand how your partner feels and what is going on between the two of you, then you may be in a position to work out solutions to your problem – solutions which save your relationship. As one mother commented:

'We talk about everything: not just about CF. Sometimes the strain is boiling up but it's nothing to do with our son and the fact he's got CF. You just need to talk about everything.'

Taking a break

One of the very valuable services which may be available through the CF Trust* is respite care so you can have some time out. Taking responsibility day in day out can be very draining and it's important to recognize the point at which you need to take a break. Paula feels very strongly there should be more breaks for mothers because it can be so stressful:

'I worry about her all the time. I'm always saying "Sally have you taken your tablets. Sally have you done your breathing. Sally have you eaten your snack", and so on. All day long you've got to think about it and it's always on your mind. A few weeks back she came home from school asking if she could go on this adventure holiday, and we had to think about it and plan very carefully. I rang the Trust and they said they would pay for a physio to go with her, which would have been respite care for me. The only other time I've had a break – in ten years – was two years ago when my sister had her for a week.'

Although she never gets depressed about her situation, Chris says she does get emotional sometimes, simply because she is so tired:

'I feel as if I've had one ear open, listening, for seven years and the only time I get any sleep is when relatives are staying.'

Some parents find it very hard to take a break. It's as if they are forcing themselves to cope because they brought about this situation in the first place, as if CF is their sole responsibility. That simply isn't true, and if you have relatives and close friends you must seriously consider taking up their offers of help or even ask directly for help: sometimes people are reluctant to offer in case it sounds as if they're suggesting you can't manage. Cystic fibrosis should never be one person's responsibility: it's a family affair.

Living with uncertainty

Life expectancy for someone with CF is now 30-plus and increasing all the time. Heart-lung transplants offer the potential to extend life still further for some people. There is also, of course, a very real prospect that children born with CF today will benefit from the great advances in gene therapy which have taken place over the past decade. These advances hold out the promise of dynamic treatments, or even a cure, perhaps within the next decade. In the meantime, though, you will live with the uncertainty experienced by thousands of other parents whose children already have CF. As one FASS worker explained:

'This is the chief anxiety among parents when they first find out about CF: how long will my child live? But you just have to take each day as it comes.'

Time and again doctors have been proved wrong when they've put limits on a child's life, as these parents explain:

'Our GP told us when they were babies that they had just a couple of years to live. Now they're 29 and 25.' (Susan, mother of Peter and John)

'We were never given a prognosis, but at the time (23 years ago) the average survival was quoted as 12 years. He's now 25.' (David, father of Andrew)

'When Kate and Jo were diagnosed after Jo was born in 1972 (17 months after Kate's arrival) we were told that they were unlikely to reach their eleventh birthdays. When that day came, we were told they were unlikely to reach 'adulthood' – which we assumed meant the age of 18. When they were 18, they both set off travelling. After that they went to their chosen universities before tackling the world of work, and now they're in their late 20s.' (Anne, mother of Kate and Jo)

The possibility of death is something that will never leave you entirely. As one parent explained, it's really hard to accept when:

'On the one hand they say how lucky he was to be born now when treatments are so good, but – be careful – he could take a turn for the worse.'

But as Margaret, the mother of a grown-up son with CF, comments:

'We could all be run over by a bus tomorrow. I just take it as it comes and think whatever we have is a bonus.'

In a way, you don't have a choice: you have to get on with life and living, for the sake of your child as well as any other children, your partner and yourself. That doesn't mean you have constantly to grit your teeth and always present a bright face to the world. You have every right to feel angry, depressed and anxious at times – but the important thing is not to let these feelings swamp you. If you start to feel swamped then you need to act quickly to find someone to talk to, someone who will listen uncritically so you can let it all out.

Thinking about the future

It is inevitable that from time to time you will catch yourself thinking about the future – your future, as well as your child's. If this is your only child you may wonder what it means in terms of grandchildren. The fact is that women with CF are able to have babies, although pregnancy puts a great strain on their bodies. The vast majority of men with CF, however, are not able to father a child normally although new advances may help some (see chapter 8).

More children?

Whether the child diagnosed as having CF is your first, second, third or fourth, the question of more children is a big one. You should have the chance to speak to a genetic counsellor who can explain in detail how CF is inherited (see chapter 1), but essentially the message is quite simple: each time you are pregnant as a couple, there is a one-in-four chance the baby will have CF.

Of course, doctors can now test an unborn baby for CF at a stage when it is possible to have the pregnancy terminated. The testing is normally done when a woman is around 10–12 weeks pregnant, using a technique called chorionic villus sampling (CVS). A tiny piece of the developing placenta is removed and sent for analysis. The developing placenta contains the same chromosomes as the baby, so the analysis will show whether the baby has a pair of CF genes and will therefore have CF. The test itself isn't without risk: there is a 1–2 per cent chance of a miscarriage, so it should only be recommended for couples who would consider having an abortion if the baby did have CF or another chromosome problem.

This kind of prenatal diagnosis can also be done on a sample of blood taken from the umbilical cord, or during an amniocentesis test in which some of the amniotic fluid surrounding the baby is drawn off and analysed. The fluid contains cells shed from the baby's skin and every cell contains a complete set of the baby's DNA. The risk of miscarriage is lower with amniocentesis, but the test usually isn't done until later in pregnancy – around 16–20 weeks. Although it is still possible to have an abortion at this stage, some couples find the thought of this more distressing: the pregnancy may have started to show, the baby movements may have been felt, and the whole thing is more real.

People have very different attitudes to abortion and you may find your own attitude has changed one way or the other as a result of your experience. Your partner's view may also have changed.

The single most important thing you can do is to talk to your partner. There are three key questions to get you started:

- How do you feel about having another baby?
- How does your partner feel?
- Do you agree about antenatal testing and abortion?

'I'd love another child. I always wanted three, although two is enough, even without CF, and we'd settled for two – a boy and a girl. But when he was diagnosed I kept thinking I didn't want an only child. Even when he's in hospital I think who has she got to play with at home? If I did get pregnant I'd have an amnio and then have an abortion if the baby was CF: I don't think it would be fair on any of us to have another child with CF. But my husband says no. He's thinking of what it would put me through to have an abortion, and I can understand that. It's not a problem between us, but I can't say "No more" at this point. I'm just hanging on, I don't know how long for.' (Karen, mother of Robert aged four)

'There was no screening available when our second son was born – 25 years ago – but we thought we'd have more of a balanced family if we had another child, so we went ahead, even though we knew there was a one-in-four risk. And he did have CF, but we managed. I think in some ways it helped the boys, having each other. But we waited until screening was introduced – another 12 years – before we tried again and this time we had CVS. We had to explain to the boys that we would have a termination this time if necessary because we were older and wouldn't be able to cope so well. We were worried they would think we wouldn't have had them if we'd had screening back then – which wasn't the case – but they were brilliant about it and it turned out the baby didn't have CF.' (Susan, mother of Peter and John, adults with CF)

'I got remarried about 18 months after I split up from my first husband. My second husband wasn't tested to see if he was a carrier until we decided we'd like to have a baby. He wasn't a carrier so we went ahead, but we agreed we wouldn't have tried if he was.' (Paula, mother of Sally aged ten)

Don't assume you know how your partner feels unless you have discussed it recently. If you can't agree, or you find it difficult to discuss without arguing or getting emotional, it might be worth talking to a Relate* counsellor. Knowing that you disagree about something so fundamental will put a great strain on your relationship at a time when you really need to be working together and supporting each other more than ever. Although one of you may change your mind over time, it is easy to get into an entrenched position and feel bitter and resentful towards your partner. It is also likely to make sex very difficult.

Diagnosing CF before pregnancy
Couples having IVF (*in vitro* fertilization – the test-tube baby technique) may be able to take advantage of a relatively new technique called pre-implantation diagnosis. This is used to check that the embryo created from the sperm and egg outside the womb is healthy. The technique involves taking a single cell from the young embryo which then goes on to develop normally. The DNA in the cell can be tested just like any other DNA to check for the presence of the faulty CF gene. If the gene is there, doctors can select only the non-CF embryos to place in the womb. Some couples may find this

---

more acceptable than the idea of waiting for chorionic villus sampling or amniocentesis and then contemplating a termination. Of course, there are no guarantees with IVF: success rates aren't high and it is very expensive.

How you feel isn't necessarily governed by the size or completeness of your family. Even if they had originally planned to have more children, some people are appalled by the idea of taking a risk that another child could have CF and cannot even consider the thought of abortion. Others who weren't planning on having any more children, like Judy, can end up having very mixed feelings:

'When Ellen was born we said that's enough: we've got a boy and a girl. Then we found out she had CF, and they said "If you have another child there's a one-in-four chance they'd have CF", and we felt the option had been taken away. Even though we didn't want another one I felt cheated.'

It doesn't help to be told this is irrational. It's a feeling, not a logical position, and as such it's very real to you. Even in circumstances where a family is complete, some people find the urge to have another child unbearable. It's as if they long to make up for what has happened in some way. In many ways this is another bereavement – what you've lost, in your own mind, is the opportunity to have another child. You may need to grieve this loss separately. Acknowledging it and talking about it is the first step. If you find you need help to come to terms with your loss then you could speak to the psychologist in the specialist CF team looking after your child's care.

If you do decide to go ahead and have another baby then ask your GP or the consultant in charge of your child's care to refer you to an obstetrician so you have an early opportunity to discuss what antenatal tests are available in your area and whether you would like to have them done. Tell your doctor as soon as you realize you are pregnant so that the test can be set up quickly.

Who can help?
The Family and Adult Support Service (FASS) offered by the Cystic Fibrosis Trust* can be absolutely invaluable in getting to grips with some of the situations now facing you as a couple and as a family. The FASS is staffed by full-time workers and volunteers

who have been recruited and trained carefully. Many of them are themselves parents or grandparents of children with CF so they have a great understanding of some of the issues you are still coming to terms with. Although the FASS is based at the Trust's headquarters in Kent, there are Family Support Workers all over the country who are willing to visit you at home, talk over the phone or meet somewhere to chat about the things that are bothering you. They can also advise on getting state benefits and give you information about anything from foreign travel insurance to consumer rights.

One of the doctors or nurses has probably already suggested that you contact the CF Trust* for information and local contacts. The local FASS worker will only make contact directly with you if you have given your permission. The offer of help is there; whether you accept it now, in two weeks' time or never is entirely up to you.

'It really helped to know someone was there that we could call at any time – someone who'd been through the same kinds of things. You still have to cope with it yourself but it's for reassurance really – just to hear someone say "We've lived through that".' (Karen, mother of Robert aged four)

Your Family Support Worker may well become a friend for life – helping you through the early days when you are still coming to terms with the diagnosis, the times when your toddler won't eat, and the day when your teenager refuses to do her physio and wants to give up on school and run away from home.

There may also be a local support group in your area, perhaps attached to the hospital, as Angela remembers:

'The health visitor put me in touch with the support group, but for the first few months it was completely above us. The doctor was there and the physio and everyone was talking about polyps, IVs and pseudomonas, and I was thinking "Oh my good God". It was really frightening. But gradually we got into it and found it really helpful. You do need a lot of support and it really helps to know people you can ring up who've been through it already. I'll ring one of the women in the group with a situation and she'll say "Oh yes, I know that one".'

Going back to work after maternity leave

If your child has been diagnosed as a baby you may have been planning to go back to work after the birth. Should CF get in the way of those plans? Julie found herself in this situation when her six-month-old son Daniel was diagnosed as having CF during the last week of her maternity leave:

'We'd had a nanny for about two or three years for my older son and we basically couldn't afford to keep her on if I didn't go back to work. So I asked her to think whether she could take Daniel on and fortunately she said yes. If she'd said no, I couldn't have come back. In some ways I think going back to work got me over those first horrendous weeks. Even so I felt enormous guilt. It's difficult enough coming back after having a baby but coming back and having to run a department and be normal was very hard. And I don't think employers can really cope when there is a long-term problem. At one stage Daniel was in hospital a lot and I used to sleep at the hospital, come into work in the morning and then go back to visit him at lunch time. Nobody suggested having a week off and I didn't ask because I felt I had to show all over again that I could do the job.'

There are clearly three major issues: logistics and coping with emergencies, childcare, and your feelings. While all working parents have to have contingency plans to cover the times when their children are ill, parents of children with CF are likely to need more time off for this kind of thing. Depending on the type of work you do, it may be possible to negotiate reduced hours, flexitime, or a part-time contract of some kind which will give you the flexibility you need to cope with hospital admissions and routine appointments. If you have time before you are due to go back to work then it may be worth talking to your employer or to people in the personnel department to see what the company policy is on compassionate leave and unpaid leave.

In theory, there's no reason why a child with CF shouldn't go to a nursery or a childminder, or be cared for by a nanny – so long as the people involved are willing to be trained and will take on responsibility for giving medication and physio as necessary. But this is obviously a big responsibility and may not be practical if the carer looks after several other children. After all, there will be times when your child needs one-to-one care. It's also unrealistic to expect a childminder or nursery to look after your child if he is ill with an infection, so a nanny might be a more realistic – although often more expensive – option. With a nanny or

56

childminder you also have the opportunity to choose someone yourself, which might not be possible with a nursery where care is shared among a team. Julie has found this very useful:

'We were lucky in that the nanny we had at the time had worked with handicapped children in the past, and since then we've trained up a couple of temporary nannies who've also had that kind of experience. I told the woman at the nanny agency that we needed people who were conscientious and who wouldn't be phased by medical treatment.'

As children with CF get older there's no reason why they shouldn't join in with toddler and playgroups. Playgroups which are part of the Pre-School Learning Alliance* tend to have a very positive policy of welcoming children with special needs. Many playgroups operate a system of key workers who have responsibility for particular children, so your child's needs will be assessed with the key worker who should be happy to give enzymes at break time, for example. If your child needs physio during the session you or another carer will almost certainly have to go in to help: staffing levels rarely allow for intensive one-to-one care.

Benefits for low-income families

If money is a problem for you – because you have decided not to return to work, because of unemployment, or for whatever reason – you may be able to claim some state benefits because you are looking after a child with cystic fibrosis. Your local FASS worker or the FASS staff at the Cystic Fibrosis Trust* headquarters will be able to give you up-to-date advice and help in applying for different benefits. For example, you may be able to claim Disability Living Allowance, Income Support, or a grant towards insulating your house.

5

The rest of the family

Discovering that a close blood relative has CF can be like a double body blow to teenagers and young adults who understand the possible implications. Not only do they see someone they love having to grapple with a difficult condition, but they face the prospect that they too may carry the CF gene and pass it on to their children. As you probably know, the faulty CF gene can be passed down a family for generations without anyone ever having CF, or perhaps in the past someone did have CF but it was never diagnosed properly. The question now for these relatives – uncles, aunts, brothers and sisters in particular – is, am I a carrier? If they have yet to have – or are in the middle of having – their own families then they may feel it is important to know whether they carry the gene, whether their partner carries the gene and what are the chances they could have a child with CF.

Experts estimate that around one in 25 people carry the CF gene. The vast majority of them know nothing about it, of course, because CF carriers do not show any symptoms of the condition. They do not have CF. The chances of being a carrier are obviously higher than one in 25 if someone in your family is found to be a carrier or has CF.

What are the chances of being a carrier?

This depends on which relative has CF:

Brother or sister has CF	2/3 chance
Half brother or sister has CF	1/2 chance
Nephew or niece has CF	1/2 chance

What does this mean for my children?

If you do not have CF yourself but a blood relative does, then the chances you will have a child with CF yourself depend, of course, on whether you and your partner are CF carriers. The chances of two unrelated CF carriers meeting and having children are fairly low – around one in 625. This calculation is based on the estimate that one in 25 people carry the CF gene ($1/25 \times 1/25 = 1/625$). If two people carry the gene there is a one-in-four chance that the couple's child will have CF. Overall this means that for the average couple in the street who know nothing about CF, there's roughly a one-in-2,500 chance their child will have CF ($1/625 \times 1/4 = 1/2500$).

If your brother or sister has CF then the chances you are a carrier are 2/3. If there is no history of CF in your partner's family then in theory his or her risk of being a carrier is 1/25. So the risk of you having a child with CF is $2/3 \times 1/25 \times 1/4 = 1/150$.

Things are different of course if you know for certain whether you and your partner carry the CF gene:

Both partners carry CF	1/4 risk child will have CF
	1/2 risk child will be a carrier
	1/4 chance child will neither have CF nor be a carrier
Neither partner carries CF	no risk child will have CF or be a carrier
Only one partner carries CF	1/2 chance child will be a carrier
	no risk child will have CF
	1/2 chance child will neither have CF nor be a carrier

These risks or chances apply to each pregnancy and aren't dependent in any way on what has happened with any previous children.

Who should be tested?

There's no clear-cut answer to this, or perhaps the only answer is 'Whoever wants to be'. Whether to have the test or not is a very personal decision and depends a lot on your circumstances. The quotations below show the huge variation in approach in different families:

'My sister had the test after my daughter was diagnosed and she found out she is a carrier. So then her husband had the test and he isn't. So that's okay.' (Chris, mother of Abbey aged seven)

'My brother is only 20 so he isn't thinking about having children or anything like that at the moment. But if he was going to get married I'd advise him to have the test, or ask his partner to have it.' (Judy, mother of Ellen aged seven)

'My daughter's 17 now and she's being tested to see if she's a carrier. We talked about it first but we haven't really discussed what difference it would make if she was. She could have waited until she was in a serious relationship, but why not know now? At least it won't come as a shock.' (Angela, mother of Peter aged 15)

'Our older son has never discussed finding out whether he's a carrier or not. He is in a serious relationship now but there's no need for him to know at the moment. It's difficult – a real dilemma. No time is right really.' (David, father of Andrew, an adult with CF)

'As soon as we discovered I had CF my three brothers were tested to see if they had it too. None of them did, but my parents left it up to them to be tested to see if they are carriers. None of them have had the test, although one did get married last year. It's up to them.' (Mandy, an adult with CF)

'All our brothers and sisters and their partners have been tested – and none of them are carriers. It was just us.' (Karen, mother of Robert aged four)

If your child is the only one in a large family to have CF you may find, like Karen, that you and your partner are the only carriers. Although you may be pleased that no one else faces this shock, it can leave you feeling quite isolated – as if no one in the family can identify with you. It may add to the sense of injustice you may be feeling. But would it really be any better if several of your close family were carriers? Paula is the youngest of seven children and has lots of nieces and nephews:

'After Sally was diagnosed all my brothers and sisters were tested and it turns out five of the seven of us are carriers. We've found out since that lots of my nieces and nephews are carriers as well. But CF never came up until we had Sally.'

Nothing could confirm more strongly how much CF is a matter of chance.

What does the test involve?

The test most often used to find out whether someone is carrying the CF gene is a mouthwash test. This is a very accurate, simple, quick and painless test which involves rinsing the mouth with salt water and spitting into a pot. In this way, some of the cells that line the mouth are collected and can be subjected to DNA analysis in which probes are used to search for particular genes. Occasionally a blood test is used instead of a mouthwash test but the principle of collecting cells for DNA analysis is the same. The test will detect about 85–90 per cent of CF carriers because it doesn't find all mutations (see above) so it isn't absolutely foolproof. In other words, if someone is carrying a rare mutation of the gene it wouldn't be picked up.

Grandparents

For many grandparents and other close relatives, getting a diagnosis can be a relief if the child has been very ill and in and out of hospital. As one mother said of her parents:

'I think they were mostly relieved that the doctors could start treating her at last, because she'd been so ill. I think they knew she was ill perhaps more than we did because we didn't want to admit it. So they thought, it's okay, she can start getting better now. But they don't see what goes on day in day out.'

If they really understand the possible implications, however, grandparents can react in very much the same way as parents when a child is diagnosed as having CF. They too experience that acute sense of loss – the loss of the healthy grandchild they had been expecting – and that overwhelming desire to make things better somehow.

They may also enter denial (see chapter 4) when they are told the genetic basis for CF. The fact is, of course, that at least one of each set of grandparents carries the CF gene and has passed it on to the parents. The diagram below shows how this works. Some grandparents cannot cope

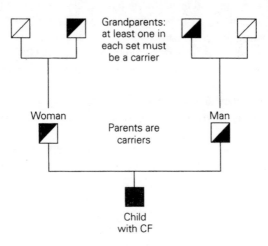

Figure 2: Diagram showing how the CF gene could be passed on from the grandparents

with this. They may refuse to accept the possibility that they could have had anything to do with it. Don't be surprised if one of your parents or in-laws says 'There's nothing like that in our family'. To a certain extent, they're right of course. It's very unlikely all the grandparents will be carriers (although they could be) and there may never have been a case of CF in the family within living memory. Nevertheless, the CF gene has been passed down over the generations. Barbara, whose grandson has CF, looked back to see if she could find a case in her family:

'We all did a lot of searching, looking back at our ancestors. Eventually I found a first cousin, way back, who died of double pneumonia, and I suspect that may be a link.'

If you have to look back this far then CF won't be mentioned since it wasn't fully recognized until the 1930s. Before that, babies weren't given the antibiotics they needed to survive. As David, whose son Andrew has CF, comments:

'We had to look back to the early 1900s before we found some ancestors who'd died of TB or consumption. Lots of babies seemed to die young as well, so you've got to wonder whether it was CF.'

Unless the grandparents are young and continuing to have children of their own there is no real need for them to be tested to determine who is a carrier. In fact, this kind of testing could be very divisive and hurtful. It's not hard to imagine a situation where, for example, the grandmother blames the grandfather for passing on the faulty gene. On the other hand, the thought of 'Who is to blame?' could haunt them, and in big families it may be important to work out which side is carrying the gene. It may help grandparents if they are able to speak to a genetic counsellor or a FASS worker who can explain the facts and help them to put the past to rest.

'I never suggested to my parents that they should be tested. They're divorced and it would have just caused another argument between them.' (Judy, mother of Ellen aged seven)

'My parents are divorced and they both decided they wanted to be tested – they wanted to know where it had come from. It turned out it was my dad and, yes, he does blame himself. When my mum found she wasn't a carrier she was relieved. But to be fair, nobody has pointed the finger since.' (Chris, mother of Abbey aged seven)

Having to consider your own parents' needs may seem like more than you can bear, added to all the other things you have to take on board at this time. But loving support from your parents and in-laws will be invaluable in the future. Some people find, in fact, that grandparents are too anxious to help and end up interfering or swamping the family with attention. If this happens to you then you may want gently to suggest that the grandparents get involved with fundraising for research into CF. They might also like to join the CF Trust* and get in touch with other grandparents.

Siblings and sibling rivalry

Until brothers and sisters are old enough to take on board the genetic implications of CF, the biggest battles – if there are any – will be behavioural. While they are younger in particular, brothers and sisters may react badly to the amount of attention which has to be given to a child with CF. With children who are younger than the CF child there may be an easy solution, as Judy discovered:

'When Ben was little we used to have to do the physio on him as well as on Ellen. We used to sit there doing one each! He's really just grown up with it and doesn't know any different. Now he thinks he's lucky he doesn't have to take all the tablets.'

Other children may develop attention-seeking behaviour or welcome coughs and colds and other illnesses which make them feel the same as their sibling. As David recalls:

'Paul had just started school when Andrew was diagnosed but when he was in his second or third year we had a spate of him fainting in assemblies. Nothing ever came of it but we did wonder, looking back, whether he was attention-seeking. Fortunately it faded out and there's never been any tension between them. They've always got on very well.'

Paula says she was devastated when the doctor discovered her younger child, George, had asthma. But George, whose big sister has CF, had quite different ideas:

'I was in tears and there he was quite pleased, saying "It's okay mum,

63

I've got asthma and Sally's got CF". I wondered after that if he was perhaps a bit jealous, deep down.'

If you have children who are older than the child with CF you may find it's easy to forget or overlook the impact it's having on them, as you struggle to come to terms with all you need to learn. On the other hand, you may be only too aware of their needs but feel you have no emotional or physical energy left to meet them. So you may feel guilty and inadequate – particularly if the non-CF child starts throwing tantrums, misbehaving at school, regressing (e.g. to bedwetting or daytime accidents) or behaving aggressively to other children. These are all classic ways that all children use from time to time – sometimes unconsciously – to get your attention. Others just fight, as Angela knows only too well:

'For Jane, it's always been a nuisance, always got in the way. She's always felt her brother was getting more attention and she's just not very sympathetic to it. He's so lazy and I do so much that I suppose I can't give her as much attention, although we do try. They fight like cat and dog.'

The first thing to realize is that this kind of thing goes on to a certain extent in all families. Sibling rivalry is as old as Cain and Abel and isn't all to do with CF. Although there are particular circumstances in your family, this may be an area where your friends and family can help – offering suggestions for how to deal with the situation. You may also find it helpful to read books like *Sibling Rivalry* by Dr Richard C. Woolfson (Thorsons 1995). Of course, you'll need to weigh up how CF fits into the equation when you consider trying things out, but don't blame CF for everything: your children are actually just being normal!

Above all else, perhaps, it's important to give your non-CF children the chance to tell you how they feel – about you, themselves, their brother or sister and what CF has done to their family life. It may take some time for the real truth to come out so you'll need to be patient. It may help to find something that you and your child can do together, just the two of you, on a regular basis. That way you reinforce the fact that this child is precious to you and build trust. Depending on the age of the child, you may need to let your defences down a bit and share a bit of how you feel, but always stressing how much you love all your children and want the best for all of them.

This isn't easy. The truth may be that you bitterly resent CF and the impact it has had on your family, but if you say this to one child it may be repeated back to the other who has CF and who may interpret the message as a rejection: you don't want me and wish you hadn't had me because I've ruined everything. This kind of declaration is intensely painful for parents and you may find yourself bending over backwards to appease everyone to avoid this ever being said. Even so, it may be there in the background and there will be times when you feel you are treading on eggshells – particularly during the early teenage years. Many adolescents seem to want to hurt their parents and can say very cruel things as part of their rebellion against authority (see chapter 6).

It may be heartbreaking to hear your non-CF children say what they really think, as Paula discovered when her ten-year-old daughter Sally went off on an adventure holiday and five-year-old Nathan had the run of the house in the mornings:

> 'He said one morning "Isn't it peaceful mum? Isn't it nice? I don't miss her at all. There's no shouting and you can talk to me." Most of the time he just accepts it, he's such a placid boy, but he does notice the tension, and sometimes I think he's trying to protect me from it. When she's shouting at me he tells her off. He says "Don't you talk to my mum like that, my mum doesn't need that".'

If tension is rising in your house then you may all need the chance to let off steam. You can use your local FASS worker, talk to parents in a local CF support group, and encourage your older children to ring the Adolescent Support Service at the CF Trust (see box on p. 68). Other ideas for coping with sibling rivalry and tensions between children are listed below:

- Look for each child's good points – skills, attributes or personality traits – things which make them individuals who are valued and valuable.
- Don't expect your children to be the same. If they enjoy the same things, that's good because they have something to share, but otherwise encourage them to find different things they particularly enjoy.
- Don't expect too much of older siblings: it may seem fair to you that they do more around the house because they are fitter, but it won't seem fair to them! When you're doling out the jobs it may be possible to get the fitter child doing the more physical chores – making beds, for example – while the child with CF tidies up books and games. There are ways of applying the 'equal but different' principle.
- If possible, take turns with your partner in doing physio so that you can both spend time with all your children.

- When your non-CF child feels unwell, don't be tempted to brush it under the carpet. It's true that with younger children in particular this may be a cry for attention, and with older children it may be an excuse to stay off school like the brother or sister with CF, but you will show you care equally if you take it seriously. Talk about the symptoms and make an appointment to see the doctor.
- Praise equally. Getting good grades at school is a fantastic achievement, whether you've had time off school with regular chest infections or not.
- Praise good behaviour. Although you may expect your children to be kind, polite and considerate, saying well done and thank you reinforces their behaviour.
- Reprimand equally. Children with CF are still children, and as such do naughty things. Don't be tempted to 'make allowances' if you don't make these for your other children.

If you're reading this as a parent of very young children, don't despair! Not only does your own family situation depend very much on the personalities involved, nobody expects you to know how to deal with ten- or 12-year-olds when your own children are two and four. Parents learn this kind of thing as they go along. On the other hand, forewarned is forearmed, and a lot of the general principles about treating children equally but different apply from a very early age. If you have a disastrous day with your children, it might help to think back over these points to see if there is anything you could have done better, or anything you could try if a similar situation arises. As Karen says:

'I do sometimes feel guilty and I think "Am I leaving Hannah out because of all the attention we give Robert?" Then I'll shout at her and think "Why did I do that?" He'll say something and I find I'm blaming her. Or they're fighting and I say "Hannah, what have you done?" You've just got to sit back and think sometimes, to make sure you're being fair.'

Thinking about the future

As they grow older and understand more fully the implications of CF, brothers and sisters may be very concerned about their own situation and need help coming to terms with the fact that their brother or sister may get very ill and die. Judy found she couldn't entirely protect her children against this, even if she had wanted to:

'They were watching *Blue Peter* one day when they were having the appeal for cystic fibrosis and Ben came and asked me straight out, "Is Ellen going to die of CF?" I said maybe, one day, but not yet, and that's why we were raising money to find a cure and that's why she needs the medicines and physio to keep her healthy.'

Children pick up on things at a surprisingly early age, so you may find you need to be careful what you say when they are around – not because you want to hide things from them but because you don't want them to half-hear and half-understand. It's usually best for children to get this kind of information as straight answers to straight questions.

Of course, it's possible that children may confide any concerns or fears they have in a teacher or grandparent rather than tell you. This can seem hurtful, particularly if you have always made a great effort to have an open and trusting relationship with all your children. But sensitive children are sometimes reluctant to burden their parents with their fears: confiding in someone else isn't necessarily a rejection of you. The most important thing is that the person they do speak to is able to listen and offer good support based on the known facts. FASS workers are happy to talk to teachers and grandparents, and you can help by making sure all the people around you and your child are aware of this service.

Alternatively, it may come back to you via the parents of a friend that your child is worried. Again it can feel hurtful that everyone seems to know about your child's feelings before you do. But if you can, try to view this as a positive sign that at least your child is talking to someone and not bottling things up.

Testing other children

When a child is diagnosed as having CF, doctors are usually keen to test any other children in the family to see if they have the condition as well. This can come as quite a shock if your other children have always been healthy.

'I knew Ellen was ill from the time she was born, but to be told that my 22-month-old son might have CF as well really hurt. In the end the sweat test showed he doesn't have it, but we don't know yet if he is a carrier.' (Judy, mother of Ellen aged seven)

Obviously it's your choice whether to have any tests done on other children. You will probably have already seen the sweat test done, so you know it isn't painful (if you haven't, then ask someone to show you the equipment and talk it through with you – also see chapter 1). But you may decide that you'd rather not know: that having one child with CF is already more than you can cope with. Or you may think that your child is so healthy that he couldn't possibly have CF. The problem here is that the milder forms of CF can be hidden for some years, but even so, early treatment may be able to prevent long-term damage to the lungs. It makes sense to talk through your options with the doctors and others involved in your child's care. Maybe you will decide not to have your older children tested until and unless they show signs of an infection or any other symptoms of CF.

What support is available for teenagers?

The Adolescent Support Service at the CF Trust was set up to provide advice, support and information to people with CF aged 12–18. Recently its remit was extended to include support for the teenage brothers and sisters of someone with CF. The services available include the CF Youthline – a free confidential helpline – which is open Monday to Friday, 3 p.m.–6 p.m. on 0800 454482.

Young people can ring just for a chat or for information. If you're a teenager reading this, you may feel as if you need to speak to someone outside the family – someone who doesn't know your mum and dad or your brother or sister – so you can really say what you think without hurting anyone's feelings or getting into a row. That's just what the helpline is there for.

Family holidays

The fact that your child has CF can impact on your planning for family holidays. Even if your child is generally well with CF then going abroad may seem risky unless you speak the language and are confident about getting care and treatment if necessary. Whenever you book a holiday you will need to think carefully about travel and cancellation insurance. In almost all cases this type of insurance excludes any pre-existing conditions. So if you had to cancel your holiday because your child fell ill, your insurance might not get you a refund. If you are offered insurance by a travel agent, it's worth making sure you read the small print. If you need help or advice, you can contact the Family and Adult Support Services at the Cystic Fibrosis Trust* head office. Staff there have a list of travel insurance specialists who provide insurance for disabled travellers. They can also give you information about the location of CF centres abroad, and about using a nebulizer on holiday.

For the sake of other brothers and sisters, it is important to keep family holidays as normal as possible. A lot of families don't go abroad until their children are older, so don't feel you are letting the side down if you stay in the UK. On the other hand, don't automatically assume you have to stay: with careful planning all sorts of trips are possible. Ask your FASS worker if you can contact other families who have ventured abroad and get some practical advice from them.

'We've always taken the view that we're no different from any other family. If it's bad weather then we get wrapped up a bit more. It's no better to stay in. We've tried to do things just as any other family would. We don't feel we've missed out: we don't know any different do we? We can't possibly say what our lives would have been like without the CF.' (David, father of Andrew, an adult with CF)

A death in the family

There's no point denying that people with cystic fibrosis do tend to die younger than people without the condition. Talking about death and bereavement is never easy and you may not want to think about it at all, which is perfectly understandable. But other people find they need to get things straight in their head, and, if so, then the information here may be helpful. Much of the information in chapter 4 on the grieving process is also relevant to a bereavement situation. When someone young dies, many people feel the loss as a great shock – even though it may have been anticipated to some extent – and as an incredible injustice. They may feel all over again the anger, resentment and guilt they felt when they first knew that the child had CF. Brothers and sisters may feel guilty they survived, that – by chance – they didn't have CF too. Aunts and uncles may suffer the guilt of feeling glad it hasn't happened to one of their children. That sense of 'There but for the grace of God . . .' will haunt everyone in the family and even in your wider network of friends. Grandparents sometimes feel cheated by death. They feel they should have been the ones to go next and are angry because the natural order of things has been disrupted, and because this is something they should never have had to go through.

But all these people may suppress their emotions to some extent because they feel the moment belongs to the grieving parents. Ultimately, everyone involved with the child needs an opportunity to talk through their feelings. There are several organizations offering bereavement counselling and support, including Cruse Bereavement Care* and Compassionate Friends*. It is often only by expressing our feelings that we are able to understand them and deal with them. In the end, it makes the pain easier to bear.

Questions and answers

My brother and his wife have just discovered that their baby has CF. What are the chances my wife and I could have a child with CF?
Your brother must be carrier of the CF gene. That means that at least one if not both of your parents carries the gene, in which case there's a one-in-two chance you carry the gene. If there is no history of CF in your wife's family then you can assume her risk of being a carrier is one in 25 (although the CF gene can be passed 'silently' through many generations). The overall risk that you might have a child with CF would then be $1/2 \times 1/25 \times 1/4 = 1/200$. But it makes sense for at least one of you to be tested.

My younger sister has CF so I was tested and we found out I am carrying the CF gene. If I have children could they have CF?
Only if your partner carries the CF gene, in which case there would be a one-in-four chance your child could have CF. If you don't know about your partner then the chances are $1/25 \times 1/4 = 1/100$.

My family situation is very complicated – who could I go to for advice about whether I should be tested or not?
The real experts are genetic counsellors. If you would like to discuss the possibility of being tested then you can contact the Genetic Service for your region of the country. The Cystic Fibrosis Trust* has an up-to-date list of all the addresses and telephone numbers.

PART TWO

Growing up

6

Growing up with cystic fibrosis

'She's only seven and most of the time she's fine, and if anyone talks about dying it goes above her head. But now and again there are tears at bedtime. She says "Why me? I'm the only one in the family with CF and you don't care." '

Answering questions

Every child is different. There is no set time when they will ask questions about the future – if they ever do. Growing up with CF from an early age means there is a growing awareness, and adults with CF often say there was no one point where they suddenly became aware of the seriousness of their condition or its possible implications. As one adult said, 'You ask me what it's like to grow up with CF, but what's it like not to?'

When children or teenagers do ask questions, it will be your decision how much or how little you say. Many parents say they never found a 'right time' and some are left with a lot of anxiety because they haven't tackled issues straight on – they simply don't know how much their children realize. You can bite the bullet and initiate a discussion, you can answer direct questions, or you can be evasive in the face of questioning. It's up to you. If you're concerned about this it may help to have a chat with the psychologist working with the specialist CF team at the hospital (see chapter 3). As a general rule, on sensitive subjects like sex and death, childcare experts suggest that parents should answer direct questions honestly but not volunteer extra information unless it is asked for. So an eight- or nine-year-old may be satisfied with a certain level of information, while a 12-year-old will badger you for more.

Susan says she never tried to conceal the facts from her two sons who have CF:

'They've never asked us any direct questions about the future although we've never hidden anything from them. When they were younger there were some fundraising posters saying not many children with CF reach adulthood and I used to point them out so we could talk about it. I'd rather that than they'd seen the ads on their own. And they're not blind: they saw other children at the hospital who were very poorly.'

What's more, she actually took the initiative at one point and volunteered what was very painful information at a relatively early age:

> 'I told them when they were only eight and 12 that they wouldn't be able to have children. I remember sitting there chatting with them while we waited for my husband to come home and for some reason it came up, and they were really upset. We were all crying and they said "We want to be like you and daddy". It was the most awful thing. When my husband came home he said "Why did you do that?" but to me it was the right time and they've thanked me for it since.'

Barbara, whose grandson has CF, believes that children may ask questions from a very early age:

> 'Children become aware of their mortality very early on. When he was only nine or ten my grandson was very frightened of dying and was asking "When am I going to die?" They do pick up on the concern around them.'

But not all children will – and then it is your decision when and whether to say anything. Paula finds that her ten-year-old daughter Sally is full of questions and anger:

> 'She knows she's got it for life but sometimes she seems to fight it. She'll say "How long have I got it for" and I say it's forever, then she says "Will I get better?" and when I say no she says "Why not?" and it just goes on and on. I try to use it to emphasize how she has to look after herself: that it can only get worse if she doesn't. Sometimes she says "How come I'm the only one in my school who's got it? George [her half brother] hasn't got it. It's very unfair and I hate having it".'

While for Angela, there was never a need to answer questions from her 15-year-old son Peter:

> 'He never asks about it and I don't say. In any case, I think there's always hope, and you've got to look on the bright side and just try to live your life.'

These days there are so many reasons to be optimistic about the future that there is much less of a sense that you need to prepare children against what might happen. Until new treatments based on gene therapy are available, the future is uncertain, but it's looking good, and it's important to reflect that when you speak to your growing children and whenever you discuss CF at home. Negative information can be used to reinforce the importance of physio, diet and medication, as Chris comments:

'She was only six when I was having problems getting her to eat. It was taking two hours to eat a meal and I was on her back the whole time about it. So I said "Abbey, the top and bottom of it is that you must eat or you'll die". I know some people would think that's cruel, but it's the truth and she didn't get upset.'

But the overall message for babies and children diagnosed nowadays is very positive and it is vital to counter any misinformation, as Paula discovered:

'Sally went to spend the day with her dad one Sunday and he told her that she couldn't have children. She's only ten and she was very upset so I had to explain to her that it wasn't true and that some women with CF do have babies. Fortunately it wasn't long before we met a woman with CF who was pregnant so Sally was able to see it wasn't true.'

Growing up with CF in the twenty-first century
Things are potentially very different for children born with CF today, so if you are reading this chapter as a parent of a baby or very young child, don't be alarmed. As you know, CF varies a lot in severity from person to person and if children stay fit and well there is every chance that they will benefit from advances in research which will bring new treatments in the not too distant future.

Explaining about CF
If you are having problems explaining about CF to your child it might be worth talking to the psychologist who will have lots of ideas for simplifying the information and presenting it in terms children can understand. Many parents explain digestive problems in terms of 'your tummy not working properly' and chest infections as 'growing little bugs on your chest'. Obviously this isn't going to be enough to satisfy an inquisitive ten-year-old but it is truthful and provides a base you can build on as your child grows up.

Late diagnosis

In a very few cases, someone can be diagnosed as having CF when they are an adult. Although this indicates that the CF is milder, the emotional impact of suddenly discovering you have a serious condition is enormous. People who discover they have CF when they are adults have already planned their lives or have clear ideas about what they'd like to achieve: in a second, the diagnosis throws all that into doubt. They do know what it is like to grow up without CF. This happened to Mandy, who is now 30. Her CF was picked up when she went for a routine medical during her application for nurse training. She was 18:

'I was devastated. The only thing I'd ever heard about CF was that people were lucky if they got to 21 – which meant I had three years to go. I'd had no real signs up to that point – only a bit of a cough in the winter from the age of 15, but nothing till then. It was a real shock. They did lots of tests, but the thing I remember most was being sent home with two carrier bags full of medication. I was just about to sit A levels and leave home and my world had just fallen apart.'

Being positive

The teenage years can sometimes be a tough time for people with CF and their families. Typical teenage rebellion may lead to a rejection of routines, while being smaller than some of your mates can impact heavily on a boy's self-confidence. On the other hand, a lot of these problems can be overcome if you have a positive attitude. As one mother said:

'Our approach has never been to say "You can't do that, you've got CF". We always say "Let's try and find a way you can do it". It's important to do the most you can: life's for living, not for sitting at home.'

This kind of positive attitude can rub off on teenagers. Essentially you are setting the tone for how you will deal with CF as a family. Susan comments that both her sons have a very positive approach to their CF:

'They never moan about it. My 25-year-old son was very ill recently and at one point he coughed for 24 hours non stop, but he refused to go to hospital, so I was fussing over him, and he suddenly said "Mum, I'm so lucky". I couldn't believe it. It's so amazing. How could anyone in that situation think they are lucky? He has no self pity at all.'

Tracey, who is 22, says her attitude to life is that 'You could get run over by a bus tomorrow'. But she agrees it's impossible to say whether she's like that because of her CF:

> 'I think it's important to live for today, but I think I would have been like that anyway. I don't think about getting ill. Of course it's hard if you lose a friend, but my mum always says "You'll be the one who lives into your 40s".'

It's a mistake to think that all teenagers with CF are alike, or that certain characteristics mark out someone with CF. But the condition can have an impact on personality. For example, people with CF can be very determined and mentally mature for their age. Determined perhaps because they are aware life could be short and they have a sense that things need to be achieved. Perhaps also because they want to prove that they can do just as well as the healthy person who hasn't had the constant battle with infection, drugs, IVs and the like. Mentally mature perhaps because to a certain extent people with CF are forced to be 'sensible' at a very early age. Their mornings and evenings are governed by a routine which they know is seriously important, and every mealtime is a reminder that they are a bit different from most other children. Even the most healthy child with CF has to get used to regular clinic visits and drug-taking on a scale that most adults would find extremely stressful. Of course there's a danger in thinking that because children seem mature for their age in this respect they are mature in all other respects – and it may take time for maturity to emerge. At ten, Paula thinks her daughter Sally is actually quite immature for her age:

> 'She doesn't seem to want to grow up because she realizes it means more responsibility. She wants to leave it all to me to worry about.'

Susan found her sons have always seemed quite fearless, although she'll never know whether this is in any way due to their CF:

> 'The older one has travelled the world and taken the most incredible risks at times. I've been absolutely terrified. When he went to Hong Kong on his own his backpack was half full of drugs. He could so easily have been mugged and had them stolen. But that's just the way

he is. He's been bungy jumping, white-water rafting and on safari in Kenya at a time when all the other tourists had been moved out because of tribal unrest! I don't think he's trying to prove anything, but they do just want to be treated like everyone else.'

Depression

Realistically, people with CF have every reason to be depressed from time to time, and depression is very common among CF adults, according to Mandy who works as a patients' advocate. When she's feeling depressed herself Mandy says she cries a lot, finds it difficult to cope with simple things, and has very low self-esteem:

'I am glad no one else in the family has CF, but you are left feeling "Why me?" My husband copes quite well and has the attitude we should enjoy what we've got, but I'm not so adjusted about the future. I'm not so much of an optimist and I worry about the future for all of us. I want to see my children grow into their teens. At times it's manageable but like everyone I suppose I have peaks and troughs, and when I'm feeling down it really gets to me. I cry a lot and I get depressed.'

As 25-year-old Andrew explains, depression can leave you isolated as friends and family find it hard to cope with the gloom:

'I think I do moan a lot – at least, I make my frustrations known. I'm the eternal pessimist, but that way at least if something goes right for you you're pleased. Talking to friends on the phone can make you feel more positive about yourself, but you get off the phone and you go down again. Mum often gets the brunt of it. I've learnt not to look forward to things too much. For example, I've got tickets for a concert soon but I don't anticipate going because I haven't been very well and I don't want to be disappointed. I can see it's frustrating for others but it's how I cope. I came to the conclusion that there are two ways of handling it. You either say "I've got CF, so what? I can do what I want. I won't bother with physio, I'll have a really good time." But then you get ill. Or you can say "I've got CF. It won't do me any good to go out to the pub every night." I suppose I deprived myself during my teenage years but I wouldn't have got this far if I hadn't. Do I ever feel sorry for myself? All the time: it's my worst attribute. One night I went out for a pizza with my brother and a friend. Then they took me back to the hospital before going out. I was up till midnight doing physio. It's bound to make you miserable and depressed isn't it?'

Coping with depression

Finding someone to talk to is probably the most important way to cope with depression. When Mandy feels depressed she talks to her husband, but she did find it helped a lot to go for counselling at one particular point:

'When I was 22 – a year after I got married – I was having difficulty accepting that I really did have CF. I thought perhaps they'd got it wrong, so I wasn't complying with the therapy and I'd started to get unwell. So I went to see a counsellor for 18 months. She was a social worker with a special interest in CF who did a lot of work with families. It was mainly me talking, but she did get me to write lots of lists – the things which were important to me, my biggest fears, and the things I wanted to achieve. Then we worked through them and talked about each one. It did help a lot and at the end I did accept the fact I had CF.'

Andrew felt that talking to a social worker helped, although it didn't change his circumstances:

'I used to talk to him regularly for about an hour at a time, about four years ago. It does help to know that someone appreciates the way you feel. I know when I've been miserable I've made others feel bad but there's nothing they can do. In the end people don't bother to ask you out, but that makes it worse. They're in a no-win situation. I suppose you just want people to acknowledge it, and that's what the social worker did. It doesn't solve anything but it gave me a chance to air my views on someone.'

Progression and complications

Diet

Adults with CF need about twice as much protein and half as many calories again as other adults, as well as extra vitamin E and vitamin K in the form of supplements. However, some studies show that as many as one in three adults with CF are malnourished. If you are losing weight – perhaps after a series of infections – and improving your diet doesn't make you put it on, then your doctor may suggest some form of tube feeding. Basically this means that a liquid diet is fed to your gut via a tube in your nose, your stomach or your small intestine. The feed is given overnight for eight to ten hours. This kind of feeding is very successful: it increases body fat and muscle mass and makes you stronger, particularly during infections. But realistically it is a short-term fix, not a long-term option: the weight gain may be lost quite quickly when feeding stops.

This is obviously a big step to take, and in a way it does represent a new phase in the progression of CF. But it won't be suggested unless you are losing weight, and you should feel much stronger and much better as a result. Although the tube in the stomach – the PEG or gastronomy – is left in place permanently, you can be taught how to insert the nasogastric tubes into your nose each night, and smaller 'button' devices are now available for stomach feeding.

Infections

The thick mucus in the lungs of CF patients attracts bacteria which produce an inflammatory response. This in turn produces more mucus and releases tissue-damaging enzymes. Given this vicious cycle it is not surprising that adults with CF start to suffer a cumulative effect from repeated infections. They also tend to get different infections to those seen in children.

Most CF adults are infected with a bacterium known as Pseudomonas aeruginosa, or P. aeruginosa, and specialist CF doctors have a lot of experience in treating this. More recently another bacterium, Burkholderia cepacia – often known as cepacia or B. cepacia – has started to cause concern among the CF community. A minority of CF patients become infected with B. cepacia but it is resistant to many antibiotics and can sometimes cause a serious, even fatal, infection. It is thought that this bacterium may be spread by normal social contact and can occur in epidemics. Because it is so infectious, people with it are often isolated in hospitals – although it doesn't cause infections in people with normal lungs or normal immunity. A survey in 1996 found that one in five adults with CF had been infected with cepacia, although another study suggests it is not quite so widespread. The good news is that new drugs are being developed all the time, so it is important that the doctors treating you are bang up to date on what is currently available.

One of the major problems with cepacia is the isolation and discrimination which results from fear of infection. Tracey, who is 22, says she can't see many of her friends because of the risk of cross-infection, and Mandy, a patients' advocate, says that people with cepacia have a raw deal:

'Where I work they simply don't get equivalent services and they're put on wards which aren't geared up to CF. What's more, they don't get invited to meetings and conferences, or, rather, they get invited, but at the bottom of the invitation it says "If you have cepacia don't come". Meanwhile, no alternative venues are offered.'

Pseudomonas aeruginosa is very common in adults with CF. One study suggests that around eight out of ten have been infected by it. If it persists for six months or more it can be very serious indeed. A new vaccine against it is currently being tested by 40 people with CF in Australia. For both these infections it is vital to get early, high-dose antibiotic treatment, possibly in hospital.

Diabetes

By the age of 25, one in three adults with CF has diabetes. The diabetes is probably the result of some insulin cells in the pancreas being destroyed. (Insulin is needed to lower the level of sugar in the blood.) But CF diabetes is not the same as the diabetes other people have – whether adults or children. In many cases it is very mild and is managed quite easily with tablets (glibenclamide or glicazide) or insulin injections. The major issue is getting enough food. Diabetics with CF need to keep up their calorie intake and tailor their tablets or insulin dose accordingly: the normal diabetic diet isn't good enough. At the same time, however, if blood sugar levels aren't controlled then chest infections are more likely.

All teenagers with CF should ideally be screened annually to check for the early signs of diabetes. The symptoms are weight loss, tiredness, excessive thirst and going to the toilet a lot – although the first two on this list are probably not very reliable indicators in people with CF. If someone with CF develops diabetes it is important to get the help and advice of staff at the CF specialist centre: the doctors in the normal diabetic clinic at the hospital may not have enough experience of what is sometimes called 'cystic fibrosis related diabetes' (CFRD).

For some people with CF, diabetes feels like the last straw: an unwanted extra complication with extra daily routines and yet more tablets to take. As Susan, the mother of two CF men, comments:

'When we found out Peter was diabetic I was devastated. To me it was just another problem and I kept thinking how are we going to cope? But he was brilliant. He said "If I can cope with CF I can cope with diabetes". To him it was just a nuisance. That's the really nice thing now they're older, they help me cope when I'm struggling. They calm me down.'

Liver

Liver complications are a relatively new thing in CF, as people with the condition are living longer. A drug treatment – ursodeoxycholic acid (UDCA) – may slow down or even stop the liver disease, but the cause of liver disease in people with CF isn't understood very well as yet and it's possible a lot of adults may suffer a liver problem without it being diagnosed.

Joint pains

Adults with CF may sometimes develop painful swollen joints, particularly in the legs, although doctors don't know yet why this happens. Non-steroidal anti-inflammatory drugs (NSAIDs) can be used to control the pain and swelling.

Osteoporosis

Although this has not been registered as a major problem for people with CF at the moment, it could become more significant as people live longer. Osteoporosis – or brittle-bone disease – is caused by a loss of bone density. There are several known risk factors for osteoporosis including low calcium intake, prolonged use of corticosteroids and vitamin D deficiency, which mean that people with CF may be more at risk, although doctors aren't really sure exactly what the connection is. It is fair to say, though, that if their diet is inadequate, people with CF may be at risk of brittle bones in later life.

Heart and lung transplants

A lung or heart-lung transplant is a major operation which is only considered when the lungs are failing. At this stage the person with CF is often dependent on oxygen delivered by a mask or nose pegs and has little energy to do even the simplest of things like getting out of bed or brushing teeth. Even eating – while oxygen is pumped via the nose – can be exhausting. When successful the operation is literally life-saving and some CF patients are still alive 12 years after having a transplant. However, the operation carries many risks – not least of all that the new organs will be rejected – and no guarantees of long-term survival. Although the new lungs do not carry the CF defect they can sometimes still get clogged with mucus, and physiotherapy may have to continue or start again after a few months or years.

Twenty-five-year-old Andrew had a double lung transplant two years ago. His father, David, describes the build-up to the operation:

'By the time he was 16 it was obvious Andrew's lungs were deteriorating. Out of the last two years at school he'd missed about a term in half-days off. The paediatrician assessed him and suggested he might need a transplant in five years' time, so he went on the 'passive list' at Papworth. It was a wait-and-see thing, but it seemed fairly inevitable because he was operating on half of one lung and a bit less of the other. Really it was never "if " but "when". I think the fact there was a certain inevitability about it helped us to be more relaxed. I did have a rotten day once when some of the implications hit me, but if you think about it all the time you'll be in tatters.'

Andrew describes how he came to be reconciled to the need for a transplant:

'I don't think it was as hard for me as for everyone else actually. From the age of 14 or so I knew I'd either die or need a transplant. I'd had several friends die and you can't help thinking "This is me in a couple of years' time". So I made a conscious decision that this wasn't going to happen. I'd always been ill and hadn't been able to enjoy myself as much as other people so I decided to have a positive attitude preparing for the operation. If I was going to have it then it was going to work.'

Even if you do make the huge decision that you need a transplant you are in fact only registering your name on a waiting list. There are no guarantees that a donor whose blood matches yours will be found in the short or the long term. Carrying a bleep and waiting for a call can be very stressful, not to mention the false alarms, as David describes:

'It wasn't until our fifth call that the operation actually happened. The other four times we trekked over to Papworth and waited until they told us that further tests showed the replacement lungs weren't good enough. We were warned this could happen but you do feel, each time, "This is it". I remember one time we'd had a chicken in the oven for half an hour and we had to take it over to a neighbour's to finish off! On the fifth occasion it was snowing and it took us ages to get there but even so we sat around for another couple of hours until they gave us the go ahead. Andrew said "Okay, fine, see you then" and went. The operation took about five hours and then he was in ICU for about 36 hours. We were nervous wrecks waiting, but you just needed to concentrate and keep your mind busy – and they did come in to give us updates a couple of times.'

83

Recovering from a transplant takes time: it isn't an instant fix in the vast majority of cases. Although Andrew was out of ICU within 36 hours it took several weeks before initial problems were resolved:

'Then I felt so much better. I was going to the gym three times a week and cycling everywhere, and seven months later I was the fittest I'd ever been. The first ten months were brilliant. But I lost track a bit then. I think people were saying "What are you going to do now you've had the transplant?" and I started thinking I should do something. Even though I wasn't very keen I applied for a job and within nine months of the transplant I was working after five years of doing nothing – and it was way too soon. No matter how fit you feel, it's a social fitness. I could choose when to do things and take breaks when I wanted to. Once I was at work I had to concentrate all the time and it was really tiring. After six weeks I had a cold, I'd stopped going to the gym, I wasn't socializing at all and they told me at the hospital I'd got glandular fever. It really knocked me back, and the last year has been really awful, although having said that, I'm nowhere near as ill as I was before the transplant. I felt so fit. It's so frustrating to know it's there.'

That pressure to have a 'new life' can be enormous. As a result of his experience, Andrew found he had to set his sights more realistically:

'After the transplant I thought I could plan the future, get a job, get an apartment and all that. Now the long-term plan is this year or next year. Even things in the short term I say "hopefully . . .". Nothing is certain. You've got to pace yourself.'

Other people say that although they are aware that the transplant offers an extension to life rather than a new life, there's no way they wouldn't have taken that offer: to feel fit and well and healthy after such a long time is wonderful.

Adolescence

Whether you're a teenager or a parent, adolescence is often a turbulent time with confusing and conflicting emotions and teenagers rejecting anything that smacks of routine, responsibility or authority. This is inevitably a distressing and worrying time for parents, but most survive by persuading themselves it is just a phase and waiting for things to calm down. But when a teenager has CF the implications of rebellion are obviously more serious. Neglecting physiotherapy and failing to eat properly can lead to irreversible lung damage and serious weight loss. Tracey, now 22, recalls how she went through a rebellious phase when she was about 13:

> 'I had lots of rows with my parents and I wasn't complying with my treatment. I used to shout "It's your fault, you gave it to me", and mum used to start crying. I don't think I knew how much I was hurting her – well you don't when you're that age, do you?'

Andrew recalls how a friend of his rejected everything to do with CF and tried to ignore her condition:

> 'She just said "Hang this, I'm going to have a good time". She went off clubbing every night and ended up really ill. After that she realized she had to take it easy. You've got to pace yourself.'

But being told you have to pace yourself is not what most teenagers want to hear, and it's not a message they're likely to take on board without direct or indirect experience of the problems that can result from neglecting to look after yourself. Hearing the message is not the same as appreciating it. As parents you may feel completely powerless as you watch your children apparently undo all the years of hard work which have helped them to stay healthy. Or you may rant and rave, impose discipline and end up alienating your child. This is a time when it may really help to speak to other parents who have been through the same sorts of situations. Tracey has this advice:

> 'I'd say you just have to ride with it and they'll grow out of it in the end. If you go on at them they'll get worse. You can show them and tell them they need the treatment, but you can't force them to do it. You've probably got to let them get a bit ill and a bit scared and then they'll wake up.'

Of course, every child is different. You may find your child actually doesn't want to join in with the rough and tumble of adolescent antics. Although part of you may be pleased about this, another part of you may be disappointed, simply because it doesn't seem normal. As Angela, mother of Peter aged 15, commented:

'He's not doing the normal things lads his age do, like paper rounds, socializing, going to clubs, getting drunk and playing football in all weathers, coming home covered in mud. Well I don't really want him to do those things and he seems to be okay about it, but I still think he's missing out.'

There are two separate issues here. The first is to ask what's 'normal'? Not all teenagers go out to clubs every weekend and get drunk at the first chance, whether they've got CF or not. It's quite 'normal' to stay in on Saturday nights and only to have friends of the same sex. The second is to ask who's disappointed here? Is it the parent or the child? If teenagers feel left out and unable to join in for physical reasons, then you may be able to help by boosting their confidence. Sometimes living with CF can be like living with a time bomb, and your child is bound to be affected by the attention and concern you are constantly showing. Your teenager may simply need you to loosen up a bit and show you are confident things will be okay. Or is it you, the parent, who is disappointed that your child isn't one of the crowd, growing ever more independent of you? Sharing your feelings with other CF parents or your FASS worker may help to reassure you about the future. Being a parent is rarely easy.

It may also help if you think now about the atmosphere you are creating in your home. A recent survey found that young people with CF were more likely to stick to their treatment if their family life was organized. Organized families were more likely to have close relationships and to speak openly to each other. This openness and closeness in turn made young people more optimistic.

Delayed puberty

Both girls and boys with CF may find puberty is delayed by about two years, as is the growth spurt that precedes puberty. This is a direct result of CF, which is holding back physical development. Puberty is often delayed in children who are underweight. This can be very hard for teenagers who want to be like everyone else – to grow breasts or chest hair or whatever it is that seems terribly significant and grown up. It happens eventually, but in the meantime it may help to talk to one of the team at the specialist centre or to get in contact with other teenagers with CF who are either in the same position or who have coped with these difficult years and come through.

Fertility and contraception

As children with CF grow up and become sexually aware it's important to appreciate two key facts:

- girls with CF can get pregnant;
- boys with CF are almost always infertile.

This is a very harsh reality for boys and their parents to accept, but the fact is that CF prevents the normal development of the vas deferens in the male reproductive system. As a result 95–98 per cent of men with CF have no live sperm in their ejaculate. This has no physical implications for their sex drive or ability to have sex whatsoever – they aren't impotent – but it does mean they can't make a woman pregnant through sex. This can have emotional implications, although it isn't easy to say exactly what causes the problems. As Barbara comments:

> 'As my grandson has got older he has found it harder to make relationships. He feels girls don't fancy him. I think you just feel you're different, and his parents won't talk to him about sterility. It just isn't mentioned, even though there may be things that can be done.'

Advances in diet and treatment regimes mean there's no reason why boys born with CF should be any different to look at. As Susan comments of her two grown-up sons:

> 'They're both very attractive boys to look at and they're very kind, so they've never had problems forming relationships with women. Peter has always been average height and build. John is smaller but as a result he concentrates on weight training and is very fit-looking.'

These days it is also possible that men with CF could father a child using assisted conception techniques. Chapter 8 has more details about this.

Although girls with CF can get pregnant, their fertility may be reduced because of changes to the mucus around the cervix (thick mucus can act as a barrier to sperm), or because their periods have either stopped or not started. This 'amenorrhoea' is the body's reaction to a lack of nutrients and can happen to any girls when they diet or when they suffer from anorexia nervosa. In effect, some of the body's systems shut down to preserve nutrients for other places where they are needed more urgently.

Even if you don't have periods at the moment, however, it makes sense to use contraception if you want to avoid getting pregnant: basically you could start at any time and you will ovulate – release an egg which could be fertilized – before your first period comes. Using condoms will also protect you against sexually transmitted diseases including HIV, the virus that can lead to AIDS. See chapter 8 for more details of pregnancy for women with CF.

> The Cystic Fibrosis Trust* produces a special guide written for young people, called *Growing Up with Cystic Fibrosis*. It is reassuring, encouraging, honest and practical. Although as a parent you're unlikely to get any thanks for it, your child might actually appreciate having a copy. Growing up can be very lonely at times. Growing up with a long-term condition, more so.

7

Letting go and moving on

'She's away at university now and I know she's not looking after herself. Sometimes I just want to bring her home and put her in a bubble.'

'Now he's 15 I know he should really be doing it all himself, but he's lazy – and I like to know it's been done properly. So I do the morning and my husband does the afternoon. But he can do it himself. It does him good to get away as he gets more independent. I try not to be overprotective but I probably am a bit sometimes.'

Allowing teenagers and young adults to take responsibility for their own lives is an important part of being a parent. You may find you are constantly having to bite your tongue to stop yourself reminding (nagging) your child to do physio, take medication, take care and so on. This may be a time when you need a lot of emotional support from people who have already been through this.

Susan feels that she has handed over responsibility to her two grown-up sons:

'They're adults now and we just can't get involved like we used to. We let them make their own decisions, and they're different personalities so they make different decisions. We've always been a close family and they'll talk to us if they want to. We have to leave it at that.'

Allowing your children to be independent and make their own decisions is not the same as abdicating responsibility, although you may feel guilty and keep questioning whether you are doing the right thing. You may also be constantly anxious. On some occasions – despite letting go – you may feel you need to intervene, although there's obviously a fine line between preserving your child's health and keeping a good relationship of trust and respect. Susan recalls one recent incident when she felt she couldn't stand back and watch any longer:

'I can't nag and go on at them all the time – especially since Peter has left home and got married. But they don't always look after themselves as much as I'd like them to. Last winter John was commuting to work

89

and didn't want to take time off to have a flu jab, so, not surprisingly, he got flu and was really quite ill. In the end I rang the Brompton [hospital] but he wrenched the phone off me and said to the nurse "I'm not ill, she's just fussing". Eventually though he did go in and they started IVs. Even so, it was lucky they hit on the right drug first time because he insisted on coming home the next day.'

Tracey, who is 22, says her parents have always been very normal about everything and haven't tried to protect her too much, but she's seen other parents who have gone to the opposite extreme:

'One of my friends with CF is 21 and she's never been down town in her life – her mum's that protective of her. She's just had her wrapped up in cotton wool since she was 15. I know she's been ill but to me she hasn't had a life. She won't even let her come to the phone because she thinks it might make her want to go out and see people. I think if your parents go round telling you you're not well then you believe it and you don't feel well. If they treat you normally then you can get on with your life.'

Leaving paediatrics

Until you are about 16 the NHS regards you as a child and your treatment will usually be directed by a paediatrician, hopefully one who specializes in cystic fibrosis. But at some time after you are 14 (but perhaps as late as 20), your care may be transferred to an adult hospital – possibly a general chest clinic at the local hospital – where you may be under the care of a respiratory physician who covers a wide range of conditions. This can be quite a shock – not only may your appointments be less frequent but you may suddenly be expected to take much more responsibility for your own treatment. Ideally, experts recommend, your new doctors should have back-up from specialists at a larger hospital, and there should be a handover year during which both teams – paediatric and respiratory – look after you jointly. In practice this joint working can be difficult to arrange, particularly if there is some distance between the two hospitals.

As an adult you would expect a team of people to be available to help with your treatment, including:

- consultant chest physician;
- back-up physician who specializes in cystic fibrosis;

- clinical nurse specialist;
- pharmacist;
- specialist physiotherapists – both in hospital and in the community;
- specialist dietician;
- social worker;
- chaplain.

Although the specialist back-up can vary from person to person, no one should be in the position where they are only being looked after by staff at a small local hospital. Research suggests that people who go to special cystic fibrosis clinics have better overall control of their symptoms. Obviously you may want to avoid travelling long distances on a regular basis, but if doctors from different centres are willing to co-operate it should be possible to get this specialist care. If you aren't satisfied with the level of care you are receiving there are a number of things you could do. You could contact the doctors in charge of your care when you were a child to see if they can sort something out; you could ask your GP to refer you to a regional specialist centre; or you could contact the Family and Adult Support Services staff at the Cystic Fibrosis Trust* to see if they can offer any suggestions about what to do in your particular circumstances. As a minimum, you should have an annual assessment at a specialist centre and possibly home visits from a cystic fibrosis nurse specialist who can help you with IV antibiotics and get other people from the team involved as necessary.

Some people find it very difficult emotionally to leave the children's hospital behind. After all, it's a place where you have grown up and where you may well have felt very secure. You may also have formed a bond with the staff whom you have got to know over a number of years. Some people are offered the choice of when to move on, and if this happens you may feel in a bit of a dilemma. It's unlikely you will have to make an instant decision, so you can take time to talk through your concerns with your social worker, a Family and Adult Support Services (FASS) worker or anyone on the team at the hospital whom you trust and like. Perhaps you could ask someone from the children's hospital to come with you when you first visit the new centre. If you do decide to switch to the adult hospital team – or such a decision is made for you – it's worth taking time to say goodbye to the people who have been looking after you for so long: they will probably miss you as much as you will miss them. It may also help if you start going to see the paediatrician on your own for a while before you transfer – to get used to the feeling of independence and so you don't have to make so many changes all at the same time.

After your move, it's important to give yourself time to adjust to any new procedures and time to build up trust in the new staff who are organizing your treatment. This kind of trust doesn't happen overnight and small mishaps – notes getting mislaid, different doctors asking you to repeat the same facts and people forgetting your name – can seem like major disasters when you're feeling vulnerable.

When young adults with CF were asked about their transition to adult care in a survey recently, the major reason for unhappiness was in-patient treatment in a ward with sick, elderly people. Unfortunately in some places there's no getting round this: the average local hospital can only reserve three or four beds for patients with cystic fibrosis and these are usually on a general ward.

Some adults with CF, by contrast, get stuck in paediatric clinics which clearly aren't appropriate for them as they get older. Mandy, a CF patients' advocate, explains that in some parts of the country there simply isn't enough provision for adults with CF:

'The care these people receive isn't appropriate but they feel trapped: if you want to stay well, you can't stop going.'

If you find yourself in this situation it's important to do some homework on what services are available in your area, and, if necessary, badger your GP to get you referred to an adult CF centre. Your local FASS worker should be able to help.

Other people may be quite happy to stay where they are. Tracey, who is 22, is still receiving all her care from the specialist paediatric hospital because, as she explains, it's the best in her area:

'There's no good adult service round here – I'd have to travel miles – and I'm very happy at the children's hospital. Sometimes they do tend to forget how old we are but they try to accommodate me on a side ward whenever they can. I'd rather that than be on a chest ward full of old people. Fortunately I'm not under any pressure to leave.'

Getting on with your GP

Although they very rarely have any specialist expertise in managing cystic fibrosis, GPs can play an important part in your treatment. Sometimes they are the gatekeepers to the medication you need because they sign repeat prescriptions. While many GPs are only too willing to help with what they recognize as a very serious condition, it's possible you may encounter problems getting your GP to prescribe the drugs you need – because of cost or because of ignorance. Once you're an adult you'll be asking for repeat prescriptions yourself, rather than through your mum and dad. You may have longed for the time when this would happen and when people would stop treating you like a child, but the reality may not be quite so easy and you may actually want your parents to continue coming with you to the surgery or to the hospital. The important thing is to get the treatment you need – and if that means a heavyweight parent getting involved then you may have to swallow your pride. Being assertive and knowing how to complain effectively are skills that you can learn from your parents!

8

An independent life

'I couldn't wait to leave home and it's been great to have so much freedom. But it's also been a lot harder than I thought.'

Adults with cystic fibrosis today are the first generation to have survived in large numbers. So just as doctors are having to get to grips with what that means in terms of treatment, it's not surprising that CF adults are encountering new situations, challenges and problems themselves – particularly with employment, fertility, and financial services such as mortgages and insurance. Things will undoubtedly change over the next ten or fifteen years, so this chapter is possibly less relevant to parents whose child has been recently diagnosed with CF than it is to teenagers or parents of teenagers with CF. On the other hand, the more people who are aware of the situations facing adults with CF, the greater the pressure for action to resolve some of the problems.

Further education

A great number of teenagers with CF go into further education. As you know by now, the condition has no impact whatsoever on intellect, although people who are very unwell with CF can miss big chunks of school or college and may need extra time to catch up. Susan recalls her younger son's experience at college:

'They've always been very healthy but the most worrying times for us were during exams – GCSEs, A levels and particularly finals at university. I was absolutely terrified then that they'd fall ill and not be able to do their best. John wouldn't tell his tutor he had CF even when he was very ill during his second year at university, so in the end one of his friends had a word. The tutor couldn't understand why John didn't want him to know – he said it would be taken into account if necessary, but John didn't want that. He didn't want to be treated differently. Fortunately he got a 2.1 which meant he could go on and do his masters.'

Jobs

If you are fit enough to work there are bound to be several questions buzzing round in your head. Will CF stop me doing what I want to do?

Should I tell prospective employers about my CF? Are they allowed to treat me differently? What would happen if I didn't say and they found out later?

A 1994 survey of adults with CF found that almost half always revealed they had CF at job interviews. Although this hadn't affected their chances of being employed at the time of the survey, overall one in three people thought they had been refused a job at some time because of their CF. Some people said the interviewer's attitude changed after CF was mentioned, others that the employer had been concerned about sick leave or thought that the job would be too demanding. A small number said that they had been sacked or that job offers had been withdrawn after CF had been revealed or after a medical. These findings were confirmed in a 1996 study in which one in five people reported they had experienced problems getting a job, while one in six had problems keeping a job – an overall total of one in four.

Tracey, who is 22, says she even found it hard to get a Saturday job:

'I used to say I'd got asthma. If you say you've got CF you've got no chance. If an employer can choose between someone who's healthy and someone who isn't then they're always going to take the person who's healthy, aren't they? The only job I could get was with the chemist because he knew me!'

Tracey now has a job working $17\frac{1}{2}$ hours a week, which she says is enough. She's also found it helpful to have a flexible job where she can work from home some of the time and fit her work around her treatment. Mandy, a patients' advocate who has CF herself, says there is a lot of discrimination in the workplace, although she found herself able to take up her chosen occupation as a nurse:

'People with CF are sometimes offered different contracts to everyone else. So, for example, an employer might say "We want to review the contract in a year since you have CF". That's just not right. I was fortunate that I could do my nurse training, and I worked full time until I had children and part time afterwards. I managed all the shifts and was able to work where I wanted to. I did have to be careful about cross-infection, but it was never a problem.'

In a time of high unemployment it is easy to feel very negative – to feel that CF represents just one more reason why an employer should choose someone else. One mother expressed her anxiety about the prospects for her teenage son who has CF, but at the same time acknowledged that sometimes you have to create your own opportunities:

> 'They've started to talk about work experience at school now and it may be difficult for him to get any because he hasn't been well and there are quite a few things he couldn't do. But he loves computers and we think maybe he could start his own business.'

The 1996 survey found that only one in four adults with CF was unemployed, although this rises to over one in three among people aged 23-plus. This confirms the finding of a study published in 1993 which found that only one in four adults with CF was unemployed because of ill health.

Do you have to tell employers you have CF?
If you are ever asked about any health problems or long-term conditions – either in interview or on an occupational health questionnaire – then you must answer truthfully. If you don't, you are considered to be in breach of trust with the employer or prospective employer.

Discrimination and ignorance

It is not only in the area of employment that adults with CF come up against the ignorance which can lead to discrimination. As the mother of two sons with CF explains, innocent encounters with the police can become complicated simply because there is still a lack of awareness among the general public:

> 'On one occasion my husband went to pick up my son from the leisure centre where he was playing squash, and while they were inside his car was broken into. They called the police who were only bothered about the tub of Creon they found in the glove compartment. My husband explained about CF but all they said was "He doesn't look as if he needs any drugs". On the other occasion my youngest son was stopped by the police and asked to take a breathalyser test. In fact he hadn't been drinking, but it was late and he drives a white racy car. He explained to the police that his breathing wasn't brilliant and that he has a lung problem, and they just said "Oh they all say that". By that time he was having something a bit like an asthma attack and they wanted to take him down to the station. It was all very intimidating and humiliating.'

Relationships

There is no reason why people with CF shouldn't have relationships like anyone else. A recent survey of adults with CF found that about one in three were either married or cohabiting (40 per cent of women and 22 per cent of men aged 20–29; 70 per cent of women and 50 per cent of men aged 30–39). But this compares to almost two in three of the adult population as a whole. Forming a long-term relationship may be difficult for you if you have a poor body image or if for you, as for many people, having a long-term relationship is tied up with the prospect of having children – a very big decision for some people with CF.

In the 1994 survey, less than one in ten of the adults who responded had children, and some of these may have been adopted. Less than one in 20 had more than one child. In 1996 a survey found that one in every two adults with CF who does not have children would like them, and most want advice which suggests that this isn't naturally forthcoming during the course of regular clinic visits.

If you want to get advice on pregnancy, speak to your own consultant and ask if you can see a consultant obstetrician as well. If you want personal advice on treatments for infertility, contact the Cystic Fibrosis Trust* who will give you details of the places where specialist treatment may be available.

Men and babies

You may have been told as a child or young teenager that you would not be able to have children because CF has made you sterile. Although it's true that the vast majority (about 95–98 per cent) of men with CF will never make a woman pregnant through sexual intercourse, the good news is that in many cases sperm production does take place and new techniques mean it may be possible for men with CF to father a child.

The technique being used at the moment involves taking healthy sperm from the head of the epididymis – the long coiled-up tube which is moulded around the testes and which stores the sperm before they travel through the vas deferens and the penis (see Figures 3 and 4). This technique is called microsurgical epididymal sperm aspiration (MESA). Sperm collected in this way are then checked, and live, healthy sperm are used to fertilize an egg and create an embryo which is then placed directly into the woman's womb where it may or may not implant (this is IVF – *in vitro* fertilization). It is important to be aware, however, that IVF has a

97

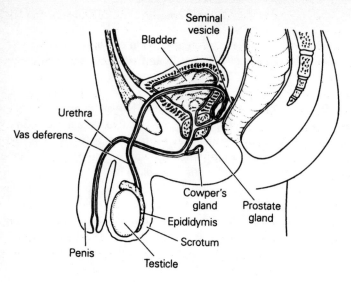

Figure 3: Male reproductive system

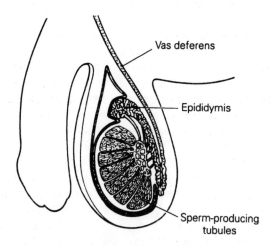

Figure 4: The testicle in section

fairly low success rate and MESA is not currently available on the NHS. Nevertheless, men with CF have become fathers using this technique.

The prospect of not having children isn't always a barrier to long-term relationships and marriage of course. As one mother commented:

> 'My son got married last year. They've gone into marriage knowing that they might not be able to have children, although they'd obviously both like them. At the moment it's not an issue for them, although things might change in the future I suppose. His wife hasn't even been screened to see if she is a carrier, although they are aware of what it all means.'

Women and babies

If you are a woman with CF and you want a baby, the good news is that many girls and women with CF are able to get pregnant, go through pregnancy successfully and give birth to healthy children. But there are potential complications which you need to be aware of and consider carefully:

- When you are pregnant your body is supporting an extra life and the placenta – the bag of blood feeding the baby – can take certain nutrients for the baby and leave you short. All women are advised to eat well in pregnancy to safeguard their own health but this is doubly important for women with CF.
- You may need to change the drugs you are taking if they will cross the placenta and present a risk to the baby.
- Changes to your metabolic rate and your respiratory system mean that lung function is reduced in pregnancy.
- As the baby grows, your womb also grows and puts upward pressure on your lungs – so that you can be quite breathless at times. It also squashes your intestine so that you aren't able to eat large amounts.
- Physiotherapy routines may need to be adjusted to take account of your changing shape and your changing needs.

Genetic counselling

Getting pregnant or having a baby is probably not something you will consider lightly, and it is worth talking it through with your doctors and possibly a genetic counsellor as well. You may decide that your partner should be tested for the CF gene: if your partner has it there is a one-in-two chance your child will have CF. Even if your partner does not have the CF gene your child will certainly be a carrier (see Figure 5 below).

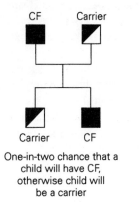

CF   Carrier

Carrier   CF

One-in-two chance that a
child will have CF,
otherwise child will
be a carrier

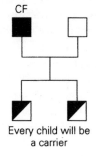

CF

Every child will be
a carrier

Figure 5: Diagrams showing how the CF gene
is passed on by a parent who has CF

Mandy was 18 when she was diagnosed as having CF. It wasn't many years later that she was wanting to get married and have a family:

'We were offered all sorts of genetic tests before we got married and were pretty sure as a result that my husband isn't a carrier. Even so, it was a huge decision to have children because we were worried it would affect my health. As it happened I had two very straightforward pregnancies and I managed with only one set of IVs [intravenous antibiotics] at home each time. It was exhausting though, particularly at the back end of pregnancy. I found I was out of breath a lot and needed a Ventolin inhaler [a small device used to deliver a drug which opens the airways]. But it wasn't too bad. I was watched very carefully all the way through by the CF team and the obstetrician.'

After the baby is born it will be important to get extra help at home with all the work a baby creates, so that your own health and physio routines don't get neglected.

Leaving home

The decision to leave home is a big one: until now your parents have always been there as back-up, there's been food in the fridge if not on the table, clean sheets in the airing cupboard and someone to help with physio

100

if it all gets a bit too much at the end of the day. On the other hand, you have your own life to live, you want to be independent and you may want to prove something to yourself and to your parents. You may feel home is claustrophobic, that your parents don't stop fussing and that you need more of your own space than the square enclosed by the four walls of your bedroom. If so, then it's worth spending some time thinking about what's involved in leaving home and getting together a plan before speaking to your parents about it. That doesn't mean it has to be all cut and dried before you broach the subject: all you're aiming to do is show them you've got a brain and you've been using it. Even if they are upset at the thought of you leaving, they may still be impressed by your maturity in thinking through the issues.

So what is there to think about?

- Your care: if you leave the area, will you still be able to get to your specialist centre? How easily? Will you need to register with a new GP (see below)?
- Where will you live? What area and what type of place? Will you aim to rent or buy? Will you share with friends or live alone? If you want to buy, how will you go about getting a mortgage (see below)?
- Finances: how will you cope financially? Will you be able to keep up rent or mortgage payments along with the cost of fuel bills, council tax, telephone, food, prescriptions, travel and your social life? (Drafting a budget is a good idea – mortgage packs from banks and building societies sometimes have a proforma you can fill in to help you with this.)
- Being ill: what will you do if you are ill for a period of time?
- Going back: how will you feel if your health deteriorates and you need to go home?

If you do have problems getting your parents to support or even go along with your decision to leave home then a specialist social worker may be able to offer advice or even talk to your parents for you.

Getting a new GP

You can get a list of local GPs from the Family Health Services Authority whose phone number you should find in the phone book. Some FHSAs keep a note of GPs who have a special interest in different conditions so it may be worth asking if anyone has a particular interest in CF or chest/respiratory medicine. Having targeted the GP practice you're interested in, you just go in with your NHS card and ask if you can be registered.

101

Unfortunately, some people with CF have found this isn't always as easy as it sounds. The bottom line is that CF treatments cost a lot and GPs have limited budgets for drugs. Fundholding GPs have limited budgets for hospital treatments as well. You may be told – directly or by implication – that you're too expensive. If that happens you have two options: you can keep trying different GPs until you get one to take you on, or you can complain to the FHSA and get them to find you a GP.

But if you want your GP to be involved, it clearly isn't enough just to get registered with any old GP. You need a good, sympathetic doctor; someone who is prepared to listen and learn about CF. Some GPs are particularly good on humility: they accept that you have lived with the condition for years, that you are the expert and that they can learn from you. Others can't bear the thought that they don't know best: avoid them if you can.

Mortgages and life insurance

Because people with CF have a reduced life expectancy, financial deals can sometimes prove difficult. This applies to mortgages and life insurance in particular. So while it should be fairly straightforward to insure your home or your car on an annual basis, it may not be quite so easy to get a pension.

The 1994 survey found that more than two out of three people with CF who had mortgages had restrictions such as higher life insurance premiums or a shorter repayment term placed on the mortgage when they took it out. One in eight people who applied had been refused (although the reasons for the refusal aren't known and may not be related to CF). Not everybody had told their mortgage lender that they had CF. A Gallop survey of 350 adults with CF in 1996 found that one in four had been refused financial cover for insurance, pensions or mortgages. In some respects it seems to be getting harder. Mandy describes how things have changed over the past ten years or so:

'Back in the 1980s it was okay getting an endowment mortgage: they couldn't wait to give them away. Now the lenders won't touch us because of me, and where they will, the premiums have quadrupled. It's really unfair: they just have this blacklist of disorders which to them represent too high a risk. But they should look at individuals, not conditions.'

However, it may be a question of shopping around and as there are literally hundreds if not thousands of different mortgages around it may be worth taking professional financial advice from someone who has experience. It may also be necessary to have a reduced term on the mortgage (say 15 years) which means that the monthly mortgage payments are likely to be higher since the normal payback time is 25 years.

Some people find they have no problems at all:

> 'Although they wouldn't give us mortgage protection in case I was ill, I have a pension and life insurance because of my work, so that covered it.' (Mark, aged 30, who recently got married)

It can help enormously if you are able to put down a sizeable deposit to avoid higher monthly payments. And these days, whether you have CF or not, it actually makes sense to get the bare bones of your mortgage offer sorted out before you go house-hunting, so you aren't left scurrying round while other people bag the house of your dreams. That way you'll also know exactly what you can afford before you look.

The Consumers' Association (*Which?* magazine) offers the following general advice on choosing an independent financial adviser:

- Ask friends (or in this case the CF Trust*) if they can recommend one.
- Look in *Yellow Pages* under 'financial advisers'.
- Call IFA Promotion (0117 971 1177) for a list of advisers.
- Check with individual advisers whether they charge a fee for the initial interview, charge fees when they start spending time on your case, or only get a commission if and when they act for you. You may well be able to get your advice free.
- Visit at least three advisers and compare the advice you're given.

Benefits

People with CF may be eligible for a wide range of benefits but the criteria are not entirely clear. The 1994 survey of CF adults found different people were receiving different combinations of Disabled Living Allowance (Mobility or Care), Income Support, Income Support Disability Premium, Income Support Severe Disability Premium, Severe Disablement Allowance, Invalid Care Allowance and Invalidity Benefit! In 1996, seven out of ten people with CF who were interviewed were currently receiving state benefits of some kind.

The Family and Adult Support Services (FASS) workers at the CF Trust* are trained to help with benefits: if you're having problems with your application or you don't know what you may be entitled to, get in contact with your local FASS worker via the CF Trust headquarters.

PART THREE

The future

9

New treatments

Treatments for CF have improved dramatically over the past 30 years or so. In your child's lifetime there are likely to be even more dramatic advances because, following the discovery of the CF gene in 1989, scientists are now in a position to work on treatments to correct the gene defect itself; they aren't limited to treating the symptoms of the condition. However, it is recognized that this will take time and researchers continue with work to improve current treatment.

This chapter outlines some of the exciting research currently underway. Unfortunately, some newspaper reports and TV or radio news items can give an inaccurate impression about the timescales involved in research or the significance of a new development or discovery. If you hear media reports about CF research it's always worth following them up with your doctor or with staff at the Cystic Fibrosis Trust*.

Gene therapy

UK researchers are at the forefront of gene therapy, and cystic fibrosis looks like being one of the first conditions to benefit from the new techniques. The aim of cystic fibrosis gene therapy is to restore normal working to the valve or pump that moves salt and water out of cells (see chapter 1). In other words, to replace the faulty CF gene with a normal copy. It sounds simple in theory but is incredibly complicated in practice. First, the gene has to be prepared, then it has to be packaged so that it can get into the correct cells and switch itself on. Initially scientists have tried two different types of packaging: viruses and liposomes.

Viruses

These naturally insert genes into cells. Until recently most studies have been done using the common cold virus – adenovirus – but unfortunately this sometimes causes inflammation. Now there are alternatives – new, modified viruses which may give better results and fewer side effects.

Liposomes

These are tiny fat particles which fuse with cell membranes and so are able to release the normal gene into the cell. UK scientists have tended to work with liposomes rather than viruses because they give equally good results without the risk of inflammation.

The world's first clinical trial using liposomes to deliver healthy genes to the noses of CF patients took place in the UK in 1995. A spray was used to get the gene into the nose. Two subsequent trials in the UK confirmed the results: in some cases and for a short period of time the genes get into cells, are switched on, and correct about a fifth of the CF abnormality.

Essentially these were safety studies which also assessed whether it was possible to produce a new working protein. The nose was chosen because it is easier to get to than the lungs and it was easier to study safety and side effects there.

But as the studies showed, the benefits were short-lived and in some cases non-existent. Further work is needed to make the treatment a realistic prospect. Researchers are now experimenting with doses to try and increase and prolong the effects. In 1997 the first clinical trial delivering liposomes and genes directly into the lungs of people with CF was completed. Again, more work is needed to assess the best dose and ways of prolonging the effects. At the moment only adults are involved in the trials.

Even if this type of gene therapy works, the dose would have to be repeated frequently, simply because cells die at a constant rate. The current form of the gene used is not capable of replicating itself and so is quickly lost. As a result, researchers are now looking into the possibility of using self-replicating forms of the gene instead.

The future of gene therapy lies in developing the current approaches and in working out ways to deliver genes to different organs, including the liver, which is increasingly troubled as people with CF get older.

To a lay person these hitches sound like insurmountable problems, but researchers are optimistic that a gene treatment could be available in the next decade.

New drug therapies

Gene assist

A 'gene assist' drug called Butyrate is being assessed to see whether it could help the faulty CF gene to make the right form of CFTR – the protein which is absent or faulty in people with CF (see chapter 1).

A helping hand for CFTR

'Ion channel' drugs (milrinone, genistein and CPX) are being tested to see if they might help switch on the CFTR that reaches the membrane but doesn't work once it gets there. Other 'synthetic chaperone' drugs (such as glycerol) are being assessed to see whether they can help to move CFTR to the cell membrane in the first place.

A cure in the womb?

Scientists working at the Ochsner Medical Foundation in New Orleans claim they have cured unborn mice of CF by injecting genes into the fluid surrounding the fetus. The gene is delivered using an adenovirus as a carrier. Apparently, the fetus breathes in the virus and swallows it. Although the disease appeared to be corrected permanently in the baby mice, the normal CFTR protein was actually only produced for a very short time. It is not clear yet why that should be so.

Protein correction

This approach looks at the other side of the faulty gene situation. It says, instead of replacing the faulty gene, let's correct the way the protein that is produced works. Several protein correcting drugs have been developed and are being assessed in mice, and then, if appropriate, in people with CF.

Alternative pore therapy

The CFTR protein controls a pore in the cell membrane through which salt and water pass. In CF, this 'pore' basically doesn't work properly. But there are other pores on the cell membrane, and some recent research has focused on the possibility of stimulating one of these pores to do the job of controlling salt and water flow. This 'alternative channel therapy' could be achieved with drugs which are currently being investigated in the United States.

Artificial chromosomes

Scientists in the United States have managed to make an artificial chromosome which seems to behave like a normal human chromosome. In future it may be possible to place the normal CFTR-producing gene onto the artificial chromosome before inserting it into the cell nucleus to bed down alongside the other chromosomes. Once there it could ensure that when cells divide they adopt the normal gene rather than the faulty one. However, there are a lot of technical problems which need to be overcome before the delivery of artificial chromosomes becomes a realistic proposition.

Alpha-l-antitrypsin and Dolly the sheep

In the last few years, sheep have been genetically engineered to produce the protein alpha-l-antitrypsin (AAT) in their milk. AAT has the potential to prevent the lung damage that results from CF. Human lungs naturally produce AAT, but only enough to clear up normal levels of the chemicals produced when the body's white cells are fighting off infections. Left alone, these chemicals – called elastase – would cause damage to the tissues themselves. People with CF have such a lot of lung inflammation and such high levels of elastase that the quantities of naturally produced AAT can't cope. The prospect of an AAT supplement could be highly significant in attempts to reduce lung damage.

The problem until recently has been producing AAT cheaply and in sufficient quantities. AAT is found in human blood but it can't be isolated in very large amounts. The genetically engineered or transgenic sheep are grown from embryos injected with fragments of human DNA containing the human AAT gene. This means they produce the AAT protein in their milk but in every other respect they are like normal sheep.

Early trials with 40 healthy volunteers showed that taking the AAT through a nebulizer was safe. A further safety study was done with 12 CF patients, each taking a single dose. Larger and longer studies are now underway to assess what impact the AAT has.

The appearance of Dolly the sheep, a clone produced from the DNA of these genetically engineered adult sheep, was significant for CF research and treatment because scientists now have the technical expertise to bypass the complicated business of breeding.

In future, in theory, it may be possible to engineer a sheep which produces CFTR.

Anti-bacterial action

Researchers have discovered that CF cells produce only small quantities of the chemicals involved in producing a natural anti-bacterial agent – nitric oxide (NO). They are now working on a theory that the lack of NO may be behind the many lung infections suffered by people with CF. If they are right then there may be a way of restoring NO levels and so preventing lung infections.

Artificial detergent for lungs

All of us have a thin layer of a natural detergent called surfactant lining our lungs. The detergent helps to fight infection. People with CF have surfactant which is low in two particular proteins, which means it doesn't work properly. The obvious solution is an artificial detergent, and scientists are now working on this possibility.

'Abbey's the best thing that ever happened to me. She's my life. She loves everything and everybody and there's not a bad bone in her body. Since having her, material things just don't bother me any more. Soon after she was diagnosed, my hairdresser said to me that she was special and that God had sent her to me because he wanted me to look after her. I'm not a religious person at all and I felt very angry about what had happened, but that made me look at it in a different way which has helped a lot. She is very, very special.'

Further information

The Cystic Fibrosis Trust
11 London Road
Bromley
Kent BR1 1BY
Telephone: 0181 464 7211
Fax: 0181 313 0472

The Cystic Fibrosis Trust was founded in 1964 and has developed into a large professional charity, not only donating money to medical and scientific research, but also acting as a support and information service for parents and people with CF through its nationwide network of Family and Adult Support Services (FASS) workers. The Trust publishes a quarterly magazine – *CF News* – and a wide range of booklets about different aspects of living with CF.

ACFA – the Association of Cystic Fibrosis Adults
11 London Road
Bromley
Kent BR1 1BY
Telephone: 0181 464 7211
Fax: 0181 313 0472

ACFA (UK) is an organization run by adults with CF for adults with CF. It aims to help adults with CF to lead their lives as fully and independently as possible. It provides a forum so that members can keep pace with improvements in treating and understanding CF, and encourages the exchange of information. ACFA also recognizes the needs of the families and friends of people with CF and provides advice, support and information for them. ACFA produces information leaflets and a quarterly magazine, and has a UK-wide network of contacts (Area Representatives), all of whom have CF.

Association of Sexual and Marital Therapists
PO Box 62
Sheffield S10 3TS

Can provide a list of local therapists.

Compassionate Friends
53 North Street
Bristol BS3 1EN
Telephone: 0117 953 9639

A group of parents who have lost a child and are willing to support and befriend parents in a similar position.

Cruse Bereavement Care
126 Sheen Road
Richmond
Surrey TW9 1UR
Telephone: 0181 940 4818
Cruse Bereavement Helpline: 0181 332 7227, open 9.30 p.m.–5 p.m., Monday to Friday

Marriage Care
1 Blythe Mews
London W14 ONW
Telephone: 0171 371 1341

National Childminding Association
8 Masons Hill
Bromley
Kent BR2 9EX
Telephone: 0181 464 6164
Information line for minders and parents: 0181 466 0200, open Monday and Tuesday
2 p.m.–4 p.m. and Thursday 1 p.m.–3 p.m.

Promotes standards and interests of childminders. Useful literature for both minders and parents, including draft contract.

Pre-School Learning Alliance
61 Kings Cross Road
London WC1X 9LL
Telephone: 0171 833 0991

RELATE
Herbert Gray College
Little Church Street
Rugby
Warwickshire CV21 3AP
Telephone: 01788 573241 (or see under RELATE or Marriage Guidance in the local telephone book)

Confidential counselling for couples or individual partners with relationship problems.

Glossary

When your child is being diagnosed or treated for CF you may hear or see written a lot of names and technical terms which you haven't come across before. Although doctors should get into the habit of explaining these fully, sometimes this doesn't happen. This glossary explains some of the terms used in relation to cystic fibrosis. Really understanding what is being said can help you and your child appreciate the significance of the treatment and cope better with the condition.

Amalyse
Pancreatic enzyme which digests carbohydrate.

Bronchospasm
Tightening of the muscles around the bronchioles in the lungs.

Gastrostomy feed
Tube-feeding into the stomach.

Ileostomy
Operation used to bypass and relieve a blockage in the intestine.

Intussusception
A condition in which part of the intestine folds in on itself.

Jejunostomy feed
Tube-feeding into the small intestine, the jejunum.

Lipase
Pancreatic enzyme which digests fat.

Meconium ileus
Obstruction of the small intestine.

Nasogastric feed
Tube-feeding via the nose.

Nebulizer
Machine which converts drugs to a fine mist so they can be inhaled using a mouthpiece or mask.

PEG
Percutaneously-inserted gastrostomy tube (see gastrostomy above).

Percussion
Tapping the chest wall with cupped hands as part of physiotherapy.

Postural drainage
Using different positions to help drain mucus in the different segments of the lungs.

Steatorrhoea
Pale, bulky, smelly, fatty faeces caused by non-digestion of fat.

Trypsin
Pancreatic enzyme which digests protein.

Index

INDEX

cystic fibrosis: adults 16, 73, 94–103; gene 4, 5, 6, 9, 14, 16, 53, 58–62, 70, 99, 107; related diabetes *see* diabetes symptoms 9; transmembrane conductance regulator *see* CFTR

cysts 10, 16

death 51, 66–7, 69–70, 73–4
defensins 11
denial 40, 44
depression 40, 44, 51, 78–9
despair 40
diabetes 13, 81
diagnosis 3, 6, 7, 8, 14–15, 39, 40, 44, 61; as an adult 3, 76
diarrhoea 7, 15, 22–3
diet 10, 20, 75, 79–82
dietary supplements *see* feeding supplements
dietician 21–3, 33
digestion 9
digestive juices 9, 22
digestive problems 10
digestive tract 6
Disability Living Allowance 31, 57, 103
disappointment 43
discrimination 80, 95–6
distal intestinal obstruction syndrome (DIOS) 11
DNA 3, 52–3, 110; analysis 60; test 7
DNase 19, 35
Dolly the sheep 109–10
dominant inheritance 4
drainage 26
drug treatment 11–12, 17, 20, 80, 82; side effects 20
duodenum 22

Education Act 29
elastase 110
employers 95
employment 94
endorphins 27
Ensure 23
enteric coated microspheres 22
enzymes 9–10, 12–13, 18, 22, 24, 28, 32
epididymis 97
equipment 26
exclusion 44
exercise 27, 29
exhaustion 44

faddy eating 20
failure 44
Family and Adult Support Services

department 29, 32–3, 45, 54–5, 57, 65, 68, 91, 103
family life 64–6, 68
fat 9–10, 24, 29
faulty gene 4, 10, 14, 53, 58, 62, 107, 109
feeding supplement 23
fertility 87, 94
financial adviser 103
financial help *see* benefits
financial services 94
flucloxacillin 18
flu jab 32, 90
foam wedges 26
formula milk 22, 24
Fortisip 23
Fortison 23
frames 26
frustration 43
further education 94

gall bladder 9
gastronomy *see* tube feeding
gender 14
gene assist 108
gene defect 6
gene therapy 3, 13, 14, 16, 50, 74, 107–8
genes 3, 4, 5, 6, 14, 42, 44, 60
genetic: counselling 99; counsellor 51, 70; disorder 3; engineering 110
genistein 108
glibenclamide 81
glicazide 81
glucagon 9
glycerol 108
GPs 33, 37–8, 54, 92–3, 101–2
grandchildren 51
grandparents 4, 45, 55, 61–3, 67, 69
grants 57
grieving 39–40, 41, 43, 54, 69
growth 23
guilt 40–2, 44, 64, 69
Guthrie heel prick test 6, 15

haemophilia 6
heart 13
heart-lung transplants *see* transplant
heel prick test *see* Guthrie
height 16, 22, 36
high calorie foods 21, 24
holidays 68–9

ileostomy 114
immunizations 17–18, 32
immunoreactive trypsin 6
impotence 87